THE

OBESITY
CODE
COOKBOOK

DR. JASON FUNG

THE
OBESITY
CODE
COOKBOOK

Recipes to Help You
Manage Your Insulin, Lose Weight,
and Improve Your Health

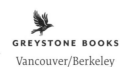

GREYSTONE BOOKS

Vancouver/Berkeley

Greystone Books Ltd.
greystonebooks.com

Cataloguing data available from Library and Archives Canada
ISBN 978-1-77164-476-1 (cloth)
ISBN 978-1-77164-477-8 (epub)

Editing by Lucy Kenward
Copyediting by Lesley Cameron
Proofreading by Jennifer Stewart
Cover and interior design by Nayeli Jimenez
Cover and interior photographs by Gabriel Cabrera,
assisted by Marley Hutchinson
Food styling by Blanka Smekal, assisted by Brianne Beaudoin

Printed and bound in Canada on ancient-forest-friendly paper by Friesens

Greystone Books gratefully acknowledges the Musqueam, Squamish,
and Tsleil-Waututh peoples on whose land our office is located.

Greystone Books thanks the Canada Council for the Arts,
the British Columbia Arts Council, the Province of British Columbia
through the Book Publishing Tax Credit, and the Government of
Canada for supporting our publishing activities.

Canadä

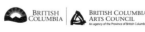

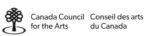

This book is dedicated to my family, who has always helped
and supported me through my journey in life. I'm blessed to have such
support. For my parents, Wing and Mui Hun Fung, Michael
and Margaret Chan, you've taught me so much. For my beautiful wife,
Mina, who means everything to me. For my children, Jonathan
and Matthew, who bring me such joy.

Contents

Introduction

====

THE OBESITY EPIDEMIC

I GREW UP in Toronto, Canada, in the early 1970s. My younger self would have been utterly shocked if someone had told me then that obesity would be a rising, unstoppable global phenomenon within only a couple of decades. Back then, there were serious Malthusian fears that the nutritional needs of the world's population would soon eclipse the world's capacity for food production and we would face mass starvation. The major environmental concern was global *cooling* due to the reflection of sunlight off dust particles in the air, which was expected to trigger the dawn of a new Ice Age.

Instead, almost fifty years later, we find ourselves facing exactly the opposite problems. Global cooling has long ceased to be a serious concern, with global warming and melting polar ice caps now dominating the news. Instead of global hunger and mass starvation, we face an obesity epidemic that is unprecedented in human history.

There are two puzzling aspects to this obesity epidemic.

First, what caused it? The fact that it is both global and relatively recent argues against an underlying genetic defect. Exercise as a leisure activity was largely unheard of in the 1970s. People just didn't sweat to the oldies in that decade. The proliferation of gyms, running clubs, and exercise studios was a 1980s phenomenon.

Second, why are we so powerless to stop it? Nobody *wants* to be fat. For more than forty years, doctors have consistently advised that following a low-fat, calorie-reduced diet is the way to stay lean. Yet the obesity epidemic has accelerated relentlessly. From 1985 to 2011, the prevalence of obesity in Canada tripled from 6 percent to 18 percent. All the available evidence shows that people were desperately trying to cut calories and fat and exercise more often. But they weren't losing weight. The only logical answer is that we didn't understand the problem. Eating too much fat and too many calories wasn't the problem, so cutting the fat and calories was not the solution. So, what causes weight gain?

In the 1990s, I graduated from the University of Toronto and the University of California, Los Angeles, as a physician and kidney specialist. I must confess that I did not have the slightest interest in the treatment of obesity. Not during medical school, residency, or specialty training, or even as I entered practice. But I wasn't alone. The same was true for just about every physician at that time who had trained in North America. Medical school taught us virtually nothing about nutrition, and even less about the treatment of obesity. There were hours and hours of lectures dedicated to the proper drugs and surgery to prescribe to patients. I was proficient in the use of hundreds of medications. I was proficient in the use of dialysis. I knew all about surgical treatments and indications. But I knew nothing about how to help people lose weight—despite the fact that the obesity epidemic was already well established and the type 2 diabetes epidemic was following closely behind, with all its health implications. Doctors just didn't care about diet. That was what dietitians were for.

But diet—and maintaining a healthy weight—is an integral part of human health. It's not just about looking good in a bikini for the summer swimming season. If only. The excess weight people were now carrying was more than an aesthetic issue—it was largely responsible for the development of type 2 diabetes and metabolic syndrome, dramatically increasing the risk of heart attacks, stroke, cancer, kidney disease, blindness, amputations, and nerve damage, among other problems. Obesity was not some peripheral topic of medicine. I was realizing that it was central to most of the diseases I was encountering as a physician—and I knew almost nothing about it.

As a kidney specialist, what I did know was that the most common cause of kidney failure, by far, was type 2 diabetes. And I treated patients with diabetes exactly as I had been trained to—the only way I knew how—with drugs like insulin and procedures like dialysis.

From experience, I knew that insulin would cause weight gain. Actually, everybody knew insulin caused weight gain. Patients were rightly concerned. "Doctor," they would say, "you've always told me to lose weight. But the insulin you gave me makes me gain so much weight. How is this helpful?" For a long time, I didn't have a good answer for them, because the truth was, it wasn't helpful.

Under my care, my patients were just not getting healthier. I was simply holding their hands as they deteriorated. They were unable to lose weight. Their type 2 diabetes progressed. Their kidney disease grew more serious. The drugs, surgeries, and procedures weren't doing any good. Why?

The root cause of the entire problem was the weight. Their obesity was causing metabolic syndrome and type 2 diabetes, which then caused all their other health problems. Yet almost the entire system of modern medicine, with its pharmacopoeia, with its nanotechnology, with all the genetic wizardry, was focused myopically on the end problems.

Nobody was treating the root cause. Even if we treated their kidney disease with dialysis, patients were still left with their obesity, type 2 diabetes, and every other obesity-related complication. *We needed to treat obesity.* Instead, we were trying to treat *the problems caused by obesity* rather than obesity itself. This was the way that I, and virtually every other doctor in North America, had been trained to practice medicine in this context. But it was not working.

Figure 1: Standard Paradigm of Medical Treatment

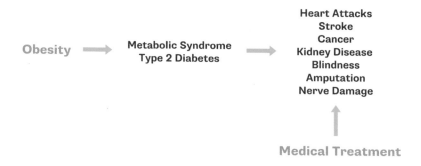

When people lose weight, their type 2 diabetes reverses course. Treating the root cause of a patient's type 2 diabetes is therefore the only logical solution to addressing this disease. If your car is leaking oil, the solution is not to buy more oil and mops to clean up the spilled oil. The solution is to find the leak and fix it. As medical professionals, we were guilty of ignoring the leak and simply mopping up the mess.

If we could treat the obesity at the beginning (see figure 1), then type 2 diabetes and metabolic syndrome could not develop. You can't develop diabetic kidney disease if you don't have diabetes. You can't develop diabetic nerve damage if you don't have diabetes. It seems so obvious with hindsight.

So, I had realized where we were going wrong. The problem was that I didn't know how to change course; I didn't know how to treat the obesity. Despite having worked for more than ten years in medicine, I found that my nutritional knowledge was rudimentary, at best. This realization sparked a decade-long odyssey and eventually led me to establish the Intensive Dietary Management (IDM) program (www.IDMprogram.com) and the Toronto Metabolic Clinic (www.torontometabolicclinic.com).

Thinking seriously about the treatment of obesity, I realized there was one singularly important question to understand: What causes weight gain? That is, what is the root cause of weight gain and obesity? The reason we never think about this crucial question is that we think we already know the answer. We think that eating too many calories causes obesity. If this were true, then the solution to weight loss would be simple: Eat fewer calories.

Figure 2: A More Effective Paradigm of Medical Treatment

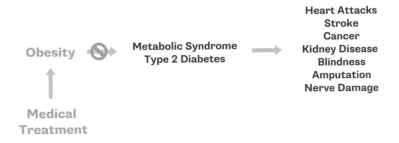

But we've done that already. Ad nauseam. For the last forty years, the only weight-loss advice has been to cut your calories and exercise more. This is the highly ineffective strategy called Eat Less, Move More. We have calorie counts on every food label. We have calorie-counting books. We have calorie-counting apps. We have calorie counters on our exercise machines. We've done everything humanly possible to count calories so that we could cut them. Has it worked? Have those pounds melted like a snowman in July? No. It sure sounds like it *should* work. But the empirical evidence, plain as a mole on the tip of your nose, is that it does *not* work.

From a human physiology standpoint, the entire calorie story collapses like a house of cards when you look closely at it. The body does not respond to "calories." There are no calorie receptors on cell surfaces. The body has no ability to know how many calories you are eating or not eating. If your body doesn't count calories, why should you? A calorie is purely a unit of energy borrowed from physics. The field of obesity medicine, desperate for some simple measure of food energy, completely ignored human physiology and turned to physics instead.

"A calorie is a calorie" soon became the statement *du jour*. It also gave rise to a question: Are all calories of food energy equally fattening? The answer to that is an emphatic *no*. One hundred calories of kale salad are not as fattening as one hundred calories of candy. One hundred calories of beans are not as fattening as one hundred calories of white bread and jam. But for the last forty years, we have believed that all calories are equally fattening.

And that's why I wrote *The Obesity Code*. In that book, I drew on what I learned over ten years of helping thousands of patients lose weight through my Intensive Dietary Management program. Nutrition is the key to metabolism, the process of breaking down food molecules to provide energy (calories) for the body and using that energy to build, maintain, and repair body tissues and allow the body to function efficiently. To answer the all-important question—what are the underlying causes of weight gain?—I started at the beginning, unraveled the calories model, and explained what's really going on: Obesity is a hormonal, not a caloric, imbalance. And what we eat and when we eat are two major influences on our ability to manage weight gain and weight loss.

Insulin

In our body, nothing happens by accident. Every single physiological process is a tight orchestration of hormonal signals. Whether our heart beats faster or slower is tightly controlled by hormones. Whether we urinate a lot or a little is tightly controlled by hormones. Whether the calories we eat are burned as energy or stored as body fat is also tightly controlled by hormones. So, the main problem in terms of obesity is not the number of calories we eat, but how they are spent. And the main hormone we need to know about is *insulin*.

Insulin is a fat-storing hormone. There's nothing wrong with that—that's simply its job. When we eat, insulin production goes up, signaling the body to store some food energy as body fat. When we don't eat, insulin production goes down, signaling the body to burn the stored energy (body fat). Higher-than-usual insulin levels tell our body to store more food energy as body fat.

Everything about human metabolism, including body weight, depends upon hormonal signaling. A critical physiological variable such as body fatness is not left up to the vagaries of daily caloric intake and exercise. If early humans were too fat, they could not easily run and catch prey, and they would be more easily caught themselves. If they were too skinny, they would not be able to survive the lean times. Body fatness is a critical determinant of species survival.

Figure 3: Weight Gain or Loss Depends Upon the Hormone Insulin

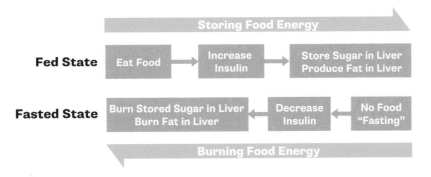

As such, we rely on hormones to precisely and tightly regulate body fat. We don't consciously control our body weight any more than we control our heart rate or body temperature. These are automatically regulated, and so is our weight. Hormones tell us we are hungry (ghrelin). Hormones tell us we are full (peptide YY, cholecystokinin). Hormones increase energy expenditure (adrenalin). Hormones shut down energy expenditure (thyroid hormone). *Obesity is a hormonal dysregulation of fat*

accumulation. We get fat because we've given our body the hormonal signal to gain body fat. The main hormonal signal is insulin, and that level goes up or down according to our diet.

Insulin levels are almost 20 percent higher in obese people compared to people within their healthy weight range, and these elevated levels are strongly correlated to important indices such as waist circumference and waist:hip ratio. Does that mean high insulin *causes* obesity?

The "insulin causes obesity" hypothesis is easily tested: If you give insulin to a random group of people, will they gain fat? The short answer is an emphatic *yes.* Patients who use insulin regularly and physicians who prescribe it already know the awful truth: the more insulin you give, the more obesity you get. Numerous studies have demonstrated this fact. Insulin causes weight gain.

The landmark 1993 Diabetes Control and Complications Trial compared a standard dose of insulin to a high dose designed to tightly control blood sugars in patients with type 1 diabetes. Large insulin doses controlled blood sugars better, but what happened to the participants' weight? Participants in the high-dose group gained, on average, 9.8 pounds (4.5 kilograms) more than participants in the standard group. More than 30 percent of the patients experienced "major" weight gain! Prior to the study, both groups were more or less equal in weight, with little obesity. The only difference between the groups was the amount of insulin administered. More insulin resulted in more weight gain.

Insulin causes obesity. As insulin levels go up, the body set weight goes up. The hypothalamus in the brain sends out hormonal signals to the body to gain weight. We become hungry and eat. If we deliberately restrict our caloric intake in response to this signal, our total energy expenditure will decrease. The result is the same: weight gain.

Once we understand that obesity is a hormonal imbalance, we can begin to treat it. Since too much insulin causes obesity, treatment demands that *we lower insulin levels.* The question is not how to balance calories but how to balance *insulin,* our main fat-storing hormone.

Insulin levels increase in two circumstances:

1. We eat more foods that stimulate insulin. Or,
2. We continue to eat the same insulin-stimulating foods, but more frequently.

Goals

The Obesity Code laid out the science behind weight gain and how to apply that knowledge to lose weight. It forms the theory behind the IDM program's many successes over the years. In this cookbook, I hope to make following the principles behind the IDM program even easier to implement in day-to-day life by providing simple, delicious recipes and meal plans.

The key to long-lasting weight control is to control the main hormone responsible, which we've established is insulin. There are no drugs to control insulin. Controlling insulin requires a change in our diet. This boils down to two simple factors: how high insulin levels are after meals, and how long they persist.

1. *What* we eat determines how high insulin spikes.
2. *When* we eat determines how persistent insulin is.

Most diets concern themselves with only the first factor and therefore fail over the long term. It is not possible to address only half the problem and achieve total success. Therefore, this is not a low-calorie diet. This is not a low-fat diet. This is not a vegetarian diet. This is not a carnivore diet. This is not even necessarily a low-carbohydrate diet. This is a diet designed to lower insulin levels because insulin is the physiological trigger of fat storage. If you want to lower fat storage, you need to lower insulin, and this can be done even with a high-carbohydrate diet.

History shows us this is true. Many traditional societies have eaten carbohydrate-based diets without suffering from rampant obesity. In the 1970s, before the obesity epidemic, the Irish were loving their potatoes.

The Asians were loving their white rice. The French were loving their bread. Even in America, as disco was sweeping the nation and *Star Wars* and *Jaws* played to packed theaters, people were eating white bread and jam. They were eating ice cream. They were eating cookies. They were *not* eating whole wheat pasta. They were *not* eating quinoa. They were *not* eating kale. They were *not* counting calories. They were *not* counting net carbs. They were *not* even really exercising much. These people were doing everything "wrong" yet, seemingly effortlessly, there was virtually no obesity. Why? The answer is simple. Come closer. Listen carefully.

They were not eating all the time.

Combining a low-insulin diet with proper meal timing is the most powerful way to control your weight. If you allow your body to spend some time in a "fasted" state, you will use the energy you stored during your "fed" state. *The Obesity Code Cookbook* offers a simple way for how to do this: The recipes in the book will all help you control your insulin levels when you're eating, and the appendix lays out a guide for how to alternate between enjoying the recipes and having fasting periods.

WHAT TO EAT

THERE ARE TWO prominent findings from all the dietary studies done over the years. First, all diets work. Second, all diets fail. What do I mean by that? Weight loss follows the same basic curve: whether it is the Mediterranean, the Atkins, or even the old-fashioned low-fat, low-calorie approach, all diets produce weight loss in the short term. However, in six to twelve months, weight loss plateaus and then the weight begins to accumulate again, despite continued dietary compliance. In the ten-year Diabetes Prevention Program, for example, there was a 15.4-pound (7-kilogram) weight loss after one year. The dreaded plateau and then weight regain followed. By the end of the study, there was no weight difference between those who were dieting and those who were not dieting.

So, all diets fail. The question is: Why do they fail? Permanent weight loss is actually a two-step process, as there is a short-term problem and a long-term problem. The hypothalamic region of the brain determines the body set weight—the fat thermostat. (For more on body set weight, see *The Obesity Code*.) Insulin moves the body set weight higher. In the short term, we can use various diets to bring our actual body weight down. However, once it falls below the body set weight, the body activates mechanisms to regain that weight—and that's the long-term problem.

It is also important to recognize that obesity is a multifactorial problem. There is no one single cause of obesity. Do calories cause obesity? Yes, partially. Do carbohydrates cause obesity? Yes, partially. Does fiber protect us from obesity? Yes, partially. Does insulin resistance cause obesity? Yes, partially. Does sugar cause obesity? Yes, partially. All these factors converge on several hormonal pathways, of which insulin is the most important, that lead to weight gain. Low-carbohydrate diets reduce insulin. Low-calorie diets restrict all foods and therefore reduce insulin levels. Paleo and low-carbohydrate, healthy fat (LCHF) diets, which are low in refined and processed foods, reduce insulin levels. Cabbage-soup diets reduce insulin. Reduced-food-reward diets reduce insulin levels.

Too often, our current model of obesity assumes it has only one single true cause, and that all others are pretenders to the throne. But multiple overlapping pathways increase insulin levels and lead to obesity. Consequently, there is more than one way to reduce insulin. For some patients, sugar or refined carbohydrates are the main problem. Low-carbohydrate diets may work best here. For others, the main problem may be insulin resistance. Changing meal timing or undertaking intermittent fasting may be most beneficial for those patients. For still others, the cortisol pathway is dominant. Stress reduction techniques or correcting sleep deprivation may be critical to them. Lack of fiber may be the critical factor for yet others. But the common theme in all cases is the hormonal imbalance of too much insulin.

Obesity is a hormonal disorder of fat regulation. Insulin is the major hormone that drives weight gain, so the rational therapy is to lower insulin levels. Most diets attack one part of the problem at a time, but we don't need to choose sides. Instead of targeting a single point in the obesity cascade, we need multiple targets and treatments. Rather than comparing a dietary strategy of, say, low calorie versus low carb, why not do both? There is no reason we can't. Here is a straightforward approach to doing just that.

Step 1: Reduce your consumption of added sugars

Sugar stimulates insulin secretion, but it is far more sinister than that. Sugar is particularly fattening because it increases insulin production both immediately and over the long term. It is composed of equal amounts of glucose and fructose, and fructose contributes directly to insulin resistance in the liver. Over time, insulin resistance leads to higher insulin levels. Carbohydrates, such as bread, potatoes, and rice, contain mostly glucose and no fructose.

Therefore, added sugars such as sucrose and high-fructose corn syrup are exceptionally fattening, far in excess of other foods. Sugar is uniquely fattening because it directly produces insulin resistance. With no redeeming nutritional qualities, added sugars should be one of the first foods to be eliminated in *any* diet.

Many natural, unprocessed whole foods contain sugar. For example, fruit contains fructose and milk contains lactose. But naturally occurring and added sugars are distinct from one another. They differ in two key respects: amount and concentration. Natural foods, with the exception of honey, contain a limited amount of sugar. For example, an apple may be sweet, but it isn't 100 percent sugar. Some processed foods that use added sugars, such as candy, are virtually 100 percent sugar.

Sugars are often added to foods during processing or cooking, which presents dieters with several potential pitfalls. First, sugar may be added in unlimited amounts. Second, sugar may be present in processed food in much higher concentrations than in natural foods. Third, sugar may be ingested by itself, which may cause people to overeat sugary treats, as there is nothing else within the food to make you feel full. There is often no dietary fiber to help offset the harmful effects. For example, you can eat the sugar contained in five apples (10 g per 100 g apple) relatively easily, but eating five apples is not so easy. Natural foods activate natural satiety mechanisms that prevent overconsumption, whereas processed foods with added sugars may not.

Read the labels on the foods you buy. Almost ubiquitous in refined and processed foods, sugar is not always labeled as such. Other names for it include sucrose, glucose, fructose, maltose, dextrose, molasses, hydrolyzed starch, honey, invert sugar, cane sugar, glucose-fructose, high-fructose corn syrup, brown sugar, corn sweetener, rice/corn/cane/maple/malt/golden/palm syrup, and agave nectar. These aliases attempt to conceal the presence of large amounts of added sugars. A popular trick is to use several of these pseudonyms on the food's label so "sugar" isn't listed as the first ingredient.

So, what can you do about dessert? The best desserts are fresh seasonal fruits, preferably locally grown. A bowl of berries or cherries with whipped cream is a delicious way to end a meal. Alternatively, a small plate of nuts and cheeses also makes for a very satisfying end to a meal, without the burden of added sugars. Most nuts are full of healthful monounsaturated fats, have little or no carbohydrates, and are high in fiber, which increases their potential health benefits. Many studies show an association between increased nut consumption and better health, including reduced risk of heart disease and diabetes. But as with any food, moderation is the key to health.

Dark chocolate with more than 70 percent cocoa, also in moderation, is a surprisingly healthy treat. The chocolate itself is made from cocoa beans and does not naturally contain sugar. (However, most milk chocolate *does* contain large amounts of sugar and should be avoided.) Dark and semisweet chocolate contain less sugar than milk or white varieties.

Dark chocolate also contains significant amounts of fiber and antioxidants such as polyphenols and flavanols. Studies on dark-chocolate consumption indicate that it may help reduce blood pressure, insulin resistance, and risk of heart disease.

Sugar, whether naturally occurring or added, is an occasional indulgence. The key word here is *occasional.* It is not to be taken every day. And don't replace sugar with artificial sweeteners, as they raise insulin as much as sugar does and are equally prone to causing obesity.

Make smart choices at every meal and skip the snacks altogether. And beware of breakfast foods. They are frequently little more than sugar in disguise, often mixed with vast quantities of highly processed carbohydrates. Breakfast cereals, particularly those that target children, are among the worst offenders. A simple rule to follow is this: Don't eat sugared breakfast cereal or snacks, like "breakfast" cookies and "energy" bars, made from it. If you must, eat cereals containing less than 1 teaspoon (4 grams) of sugar per serving. Traditional and Greek yogurts are nutritious foods. However, commercial yogurts are often made with large amounts of added sugars. A serving of commercial sweetened fruit yogurt can contain almost 8 teaspoons (31 grams) of sugar. Instead, try healthier alternatives such as oatmeal or eggs.

OATMEAL

Oatmeal is a traditional and healthy breakfast food. Whole oats and steel-cut oats are a good choice, although they require long cooking times to break down the significant amounts of fiber they contain. Avoid instant oatmeal, which is heavily processed and refined. Many instant oatmeals are flavored artificially and contain large amounts of sugar.

EGGS

A natural whole food, previously shunned due to cholesterol concerns, eggs can be enjoyed in a variety of ways. Egg whites are high in protein, and yolks contain many vitamins and minerals, including choline and selenium. Eggs are particularly good sources of lutein and zeaxanthin, antioxidants that may help protect against eye problems such as macular degeneration and cataracts. The cholesterol in eggs may change the cholesterol particles in your blood to the larger, less harmful particles. Indeed, large epidemiological studies have failed to link increased egg consumption to increased heart disease. Most of all, eat eggs because they are delicious, whole, unprocessed foods.

IF YOU ARE not hungry for breakfast, it's perfectly acceptable to break your fast at noon with a healthy lunch. But there's nothing inherently wrong with eating breakfast either. Remember, eat whole, unprocessed foods at all meals and skip the snacks. And if you don't have time to eat? Then don't eat, but don't reach for a sugar-sweetened drink instead.

The sugar-sweetened drink is one of the leading sources of added sugars in the North American diet. This includes all soda pop, sugar-sweetened teas, fruit juice, fruit punch, vitamin water, smoothies, shakes, lemonade, chocolate or other flavored milks, iced coffee drinks, and energy drinks. Hot drinks such as hot chocolate, mochaccino, and coffee and tea can also be laden with sugar, especially when you don't make them yourself at home.

What about alcohol? Alcohol is made from the fermentation of sugars and starches from various sources. Yeasts eat the sugars and convert them to alcohol. Moderate consumption of red wine does not raise insulin or impair insulin sensitivity, and therefore may be enjoyed occasionally. Up to two glasses a day (4 ounces/175 milliliters per glass) is not associated with major weight gain and may improve insulin sensitivity. But trendy alcoholic drinks such as "hard" lemonade, flavored wine coolers, cider, beer, and traditional liqueurs and cocktails are often loaded with syrups and other sweet flavorings and can add significant amounts of sugar to your diet.

What is left to drink? The best drink is really just plain or sparkling water. Slices of lemon, lime, or orange are a refreshing addition. Infusing water by adding fruits (e.g., strawberries), herbs (e.g., mint), or vegetables (e.g., cucumber) and leaving it overnight is a great way to give it some flavor. Use these infused waters with a home carbonation machine like a SodaStream to make your own flavored sparkling water for pennies a glass. Several other drinks are also delicious and do not raise insulin (see below).

COFFEE

Due to its high caffeine content, coffee is sometimes considered unhealthy. However, recent research has come to the opposite conclusion, perhaps because coffee is a major source of antioxidants, magnesium, lignans, and chlorogenic acid. Coffee, even the decaffeinated version, appears to protect against type 2 diabetes. In a 2009 review, every daily cup of coffee lowered the risk of diabetes by 7 percent—even up to six cups per day (for a reduced risk of 42 percent). Coffee may guard against Alzheimer's disease and Parkinson's disease, as well as liver cirrhosis and liver cancer. While these correlation studies are suggestive, they are not proof of benefit. However, they do suggest that coffee may not be as harmful as we had imagined. (But remember to skip the sugar!)

TEA

After water, tea is the most popular beverage in the world. Black tea is the most common variety, accounting for almost 75 percent of global tea consumption. The harvested leaves are fully fermented, giving the tea its characteristic black color. Black tea tends to be higher in caffeine than other varieties. Oolong tea is semi-fermented, meaning that it undergoes a shorter period of fermentation. Green tea is unfermented. Instead, the freshly harvested leaves are immediately steamed to stop fermentation, giving green tea a much more delicate and floral taste. Green tea is naturally much lower in caffeine than coffee, making this drink ideal for those who are sensitive to caffeine's stimulant effects.

Polyphenols in green tea may boost metabolism, which can improve fat burning. Furthermore, drinking green tea has been linked to increased fat oxidation during exercise, increased resting energy expenditure, and a lower risk of various types of cancer. Green tea is a particularly rich source of catechins, which are believed to protect against metabolic diseases. Brewing green tea does destroy some of its healthful catechins, so another good option is to use tea crystals (I like Pique tea crystals, which use cold-brew crystallization to increase the catechin content).

Herbal teas are infusions of herbs, spices, or other plant matter in hot water. These are not true teas since they do not contain tea leaves. Nevertheless, they make excellent drinks without added sugars.

BONE BROTH

Virtually every culture's culinary traditions include nutritious and delicious bone broth—bones simmered with vegetables, herbs, and spices for flavoring. The long simmering time (four to forty-eight hours) releases most of the bones' minerals, gelatin, and nutrients. The addition of a small amount of vinegar during cooking helps leach some of the stored minerals. Bone broths are very high in amino acids such as proline, arginine, and glycine, as well as minerals such as calcium, magnesium, and phosphorus.

Step 2: Reduce your consumption of refined grains

Refined grains such as white flour stimulate insulin to a greater degree than virtually any other food. If you reduce your consumption of flour and refined grains, you will substantially improve your weight-loss potential. White flour, being nutritionally bankrupt, can be safely reduced or even eliminated from your diet. Enriched white flours have had all their nutrients stripped out during processing and added back later for a veneer of healthiness.

Whole wheat and whole-grain grains and flours are a minimal improvement over white flour because they contain more vitamins and fiber, which help protect against insulin spikes. However, whole-grain flour is still highly processed in a modern flour mill. Traditional stone-mill ground flour is preferable. The ultrafine particles produced by modern milling techniques ensure rapid absorption of flour, even whole wheat flour, by the intestine, which increases the insulin effect.

Carbohydrates should be enjoyed in their natural, whole, unprocessed form. Many traditional diets built around carbohydrates cause neither poor health nor obesity. Remember: The toxicity in much Western food stems from the processing rather than the food itself. The carbohydrates in Western diets are heavily skewed toward refined grains and are thus highly obesogenic. Many unprocessed, unrefined vegetables, even root vegetables, are healthy carbohydrate-containing foods that have a relatively minor effect on insulin. Some great alternatives to refined grains are seeds and legumes.

QUINOA

Technically a seed but often used as a grain, quinoa has been referred to as "the mother of all grains." It was grown originally by the Inca in South America but is now widely available in three varieties: red, white, and black. Quinoa is very high in fiber, protein, and vitamins. In addition, it has a low glycemic index and contains plenty of antioxidants, such as quercetin and kaempferol, that are believed to be anti-inflammatory.

CHIA SEEDS

These ancient seeds are native to South and Central America and have been dated to the Aztecs and Mayans. Their name is derived from the ancient Mayan word for strength. Chia seeds, regardless of color, are high in fiber, vitamins, minerals, omega 3, proteins, and antioxidants.

BEANS

Dried beans and peas are a versatile, fiber-rich carbohydrate staple of many traditional diets and an extremely good source of protein. They come in a wide range of colors, flavors, and textures, from green lentils to black-eyed peas, and red kidney beans to dark brown chickpeas. Canned beans are also great, but be sure to rinse them well before using them.

Step 3: Moderate your protein consumption

In contrast to refined grains, food sources of protein such as meats and poultry, seafood, eggs, dairy products, nuts and seeds, and legumes cannot and should not be eliminated from your diet. But it is not advisable to eat a very high-protein diet, which is often overly reliant on egg whites, very lean meats, or processed proteins such as shakes and supplements. Instead, moderate the amount of protein in your diet to 20 to 30 percent of your total calories and aim for a variety of sources. Excessively high-protein diets can lower insulin but are often expensive to maintain and allow relatively few food choices.

Step 4: Increase your consumption of natural fats

Of the three major macronutrients (carbohydrates, proteins, and fats), dietary fat is the least likely to stimulate insulin. Thus, dietary fat is not inherently fattening but rather potentially protective. And it adds flavor to any meal. The key is to strive for a higher proportion of natural unprocessed fats, including olive oil, butter, coconut oil, beef tallow, and leaf lard. Avoid highly processed vegetable oils, including nut and seed oils, which are high in inflammatory omega 6 fatty acids and may have detrimental health effects. Instead, stock up on a few of these flavorful favorites.

OLIVE OIL

The Mediterranean diet, widely acknowledged as a healthy diet, is high in oleic acid, one of the monounsaturated fats contained in olive oil. There are different methods of extracting olive oil, and these differences are reflected in the grading. To obtain the oil, ripe olive fruit is crushed into a paste and then cold pressed. Extra virgin olive oil is extracted using these mechanical means only and is certainly the best choice. Other grades of olive oil rely on chemical methods and/or high heat to extract the oil and neutralize bad tastes and should be avoided. Be aware that "pure olive oil" often denotes these refined oils. Olive oil contains large amounts of antioxidants, including polyphenols and oleocanthal, which has anti-inflammatory properties. It is purported to reduce inflammation, lower cholesterol, decrease blood clotting, and reduce blood pressure. Together, these potential properties may reduce the overall risk of cardiovascular disease, including heart attacks and strokes.

NUTS

Prominent in the Mediterranean diet but long shunned for their high fat content, nuts are now recognized as offering significant health benefits. In addition to providing healthy fats, they are naturally high in fiber and low in carbohydrates. They may be enjoyed raw or simply toasted, but avoid those with added sugars, like honey-toasted nuts. Walnuts, in particular, are high in omega 3 fatty acids, which may be beneficial for heart health. Nut milks without added sugars are also delicious.

FULL-FAT DAIRY PRODUCTS

Milk, cream, yogurt, and cheese are delicious and can be enjoyed without concern about fattening effects. A review of twenty-nine randomized control trials showed neither a fat-gaining nor fat-reducing effect from their consumption. Full-fat dairy is associated with a 62 percent lower risk of type 2 diabetes. Choose whole-fat dairy products, and raw or organic if you prefer. All milks, including sheep's and goat's milks, are healthy.

AVOCADOS

This fruit has been recently recognized as a very healthy and delicious addition to any diet. High in vitamins and particularly high in potassium, the avocado is unique among fruits for being very low in carbohydrates and high in the monounsaturated fat oleic acid. Furthermore, it is very high in both soluble and insoluble fiber.

Step 5: Increase your consumption of fiber and vinegar

Fiber can reduce the insulin-stimulating effects of carbohydrates, making it one of the main protective factors against obesity. The average North American diet falls far short of recommended daily intake levels, however, because fiber is often removed during processing. Natural whole foods such as fruits, berries, vegetables, whole grains, flax seeds, chia seeds, beans, nuts, oatmeal, and pumpkin seeds provide ample fiber.

VINEGAR

Used in many traditional foods, vinegar—in any of its many forms—may help reduce insulin spikes when eaten with high-carbohydrate foods. For example, vinegar added to sushi rice reduces its glycemic index by between 20 and 40 percent. Similarly, fish and chips are often eaten with malt vinegar, and bread is often dipped in oil and vinegar. Try mixing apple cider vinegar in some water for a very refreshing drink. Be careful to avoid vinegars with added sugars.

What to eat to encourage weight loss:

1. Fewer added sugars
2. Fewer refined grains
3. Moderate levels of protein
4. More natural fats
5. More fiber and vinegar

WHEN TO EAT

THE DIET (What to Eat) addresses the first half of the problem, but remember that long-term weight loss is a two-factor process. *Two* major factors maintain our insulin at a high level. The first is the food we choose to eat: what we eat and how much of it is fattening. When we eat, insulin goes up and our body gets hormonal orders to store body fat. But the total insulin effect on the body is not simply determined by how high insulin levels get. It also depends critically upon how long those insulin levels stay up for. That's why it's so important to allow periods when insulin levels are allowed to drift downwards. Fasting (When to Eat) addresses the second half of the problem. Fasting corrects some of the hormonal problems that cause obesity and so helps maintain long-term weight loss. Combining the proper diet with intermittent fasting is a time-tested weight-maintenance method.

What does that mean? Suppose you spend $1,000 in one day. That's a fantastic shopping day. If this happens only once a year, that's acceptable. However, if it happens every single day, you will soon be very poor. So, the total effect depends not only upon the level but also the duration and frequency of the activity. Insulin is no different. The total insulin effect depends not only upon how high insulin levels get (which depends upon the foods we choose to eat), but also upon how persistent those high insulin levels are. This depends upon how often you eat, which is an entirely different issue than which foods we choose to eat. If you are trying to lose weight, an insulin spike once or twice a day is far preferable to multiple spikes per day.

How can we induce our body into a temporary state of very low insulin levels? Because all foods raise insulin, the only way for us to lower it is to completely abstain from eating. The answer we are looking for is, in a word, *fasting*. Fasting refers to any period in which you do not eat. This may be several hours (between meals) or several weeks. For weight loss and a reversal of type 2 diabetes, I commonly recommend intermittent fasts of sixteen to thirty-six hours.

Fasting is one of the oldest remedies in history, but it is not to be confused with starvation, which is a notably unhealthy state. Starvation is *involuntary* abstinence from food; it is neither deliberate nor controlled. If you have not eaten for a while, and have no idea when you will eat again, you are starving. By contrast, fasting is *voluntary* abstinence from food for spiritual, health, or other reasons. You may fast as long as you like, but you can always decide to eat again, if you like.

People often worry that if they don't eat, they'll have less energy and they won't be able to concentrate as well, but that's simply not true. Think about the last time you ate a huge meal—for example, at Thanksgiving. Did you feel more energetic and mentally alert afterward? Or did you feel sleepy and a little dopey? More likely the latter. Eating shunts blood to your digestive system to cope with the huge influx of food, leaving less blood for brain function. Fasting does the opposite, meaning there's more blood for your brain. The human body has adapted to function and thrive in the temporary absence of food.

Glucose and fat are our main sources of energy. When glucose is not available, the body adjusts by using fat. Fat is simply our stored food energy. That's what it's designed for. In times of food scarcity, stored food (fat) is naturally released to fuel our bodies. That's entirely normal. The transition from the fed state to the fasted state occurs in several stages:

1. **Feeding**: During meals, insulin levels go up, allowing glucose uptake by tissues such as the muscles or brain for direct use as energy. Excess glucose is stored as glycogen in the liver.

2. **The post-absorptive phase (six to twenty-four hours after fasting starts)**: Insulin levels fall. The breakdown of liver glycogen releases glucose for energy. Glycogen stores last for roughly twenty-four hours.

3. **Gluconeogenesis (twenty-four hours to two days)**: The liver manufactures new glucose from amino acids and glycerol. In people who do not have diabetes, glucose levels fall but stay within the normal range.

4. **Ketosis (one to three days after fasting starts)**: The storage form of fat, triglycerides, is broken into the glycerol backbone and three fatty acid chains. Glycerol is used for gluconeogenesis. Fatty acids may be used directly for energy by many tissues in the body, but not the brain. Ketone bodies, capable of crossing the blood-brain barrier, are produced from fatty acids for use by the brain. Ketones can supply up to 75 percent of the energy used by the brain.

5. **Protein conservation phase (after five days)**: High levels of growth hormone maintain muscle mass and lean tissues. The energy required to maintain basal metabolism is almost entirely produced by available free fatty acids and ketones. Increased norepinephrine (adrenalin) levels prevent a decrease in metabolic rate.

With fasting periods of sixteen to thirty-six hours, blood glucose levels remain normal as the body switches over to burning fat for energy. More recently, alternate daily fasting has been studied as an acceptable technique for weight loss. Here is a straightforward approach to effectively lower insulin and lose weight by managing when you eat.

Step 1: Eat only when you're hungry

Many people eat at mealtimes even if they are not hungry. For example, the common advice is to eat something, anything, as soon as you step out of bed. But breakfast needs to be downgraded from "most important meal of the day" to "meal." Remember that you will always eat breakfast. It is simply the meal that breaks your fast. Therefore, if you do not eat until 2:00 p.m., that is your "break fast" meal. Is there something magical about eating a large amount of food early in the day, even if you are not particularly hungry or inclined to eat? No. Is there a rule that says you have to eat three times a day, every day, even if you don't have an appetite? No. Eating, almost by its very definition, does not make you lose weight.

SKIP THE SNACKS

The "healthy" snack is one of the greatest weight-loss deceptions. As recently as the 1970s, most people still ate just three meals per day. By the 2000s, the "grazing is healthy" mantra had taken hold and the average American was eating five or six times per day. Even more unbelievable is that somehow we were hoodwinked into believing this was good for us! Nutritional authorities urged us to eat, eat, eat to lose weight! It *sounds* pretty stupid because it *is* pretty stupid. Constant stimulation of insulin eventually leads to insulin resistance.

Are snacks necessary? No. When you find yourself reaching for a snack, ask yourself this question: Are you really hungry, or just bored? Keep snacks completely out of sight. If you have a snack habit, replace that habit with one that is less destructive to your health. Perhaps a cup of green tea in the afternoon should be your new habit. There's a simple answer to the question of what to eat at snack time: Nothing. Don't eat snacks. Period. Simplify your life.

Step 2: Fast intermittently

One crucial aspect of fasting that differentiates it from other diets is its intermittent nature. Diets fail because of their constancy. The defining characteristic of life on Earth is homeostasis. In other words, any constant stimulus will eventually be met with an adaptation that resists the change. Persistent exposure to decreased calories results in adaptation (resistance): the body eventually responds by reducing total energy expenditure, leading to a plateau in weight loss and eventually to weight regain.

By contrast, intermittent fasting constantly shakes up our hormone production. Our diets must be *intermittent,* not steady. Food is a celebration of life. Every culture in the world celebrates with large feasts. That's normal, and it's good. Should you eat lots of food on your birthday? Absolutely. Should you eat lots of food at a wedding? Absolutely.

But follow your feasting with fasting. That's the natural cycle of life. We cannot feast all the time. We cannot fast all the time. That doesn't work.

If you haven't attempted fasting before, you may feel daunted. However, as with most things, fasting becomes easier with practice. Devout Muslims fast for one month of the year and are supposed to fast two days a week. There are an estimated 1.6 billion Muslims in the world. There are an estimated 14 million Mormons who are supposed to fast once a month. There are an estimated 350 million Buddhists, many of whom fast regularly. Almost one-third of the population of the entire world is supposed to fast routinely, according to their belief system. There is no question that it can be done.

Fasting can be combined with any diet. It makes no difference whether you don't eat meat, dairy, or gluten, you can still fast. Eating grass-fed, organic beef is healthy, but it can also be expensive. Fasting saves you money on groceries. Eating homemade, prepared-from-scratch meals is healthy, but it can also be time-consuming. Fasting saves you precious time. Life becomes simpler when you don't need to worry about planning, shopping, or preparing as many meals.

When to eat to encourage weight loss:

1. Eat only when you're hungry.
2. Fast intermittently.

We have discussed what to eat: fewer refined grains and sugars, moderate amounts of protein, and more healthy fats. Maximize your intake of protective factors such as fiber and vinegar. Choose only natural, unprocessed foods.

And now you know when to eat: Eat only when you're hungry to balance insulin-dominant periods with insulin-deficient periods, and fast intermittently to balance your feeding and fasting periods. Eating continuously is a recipe for weight gain. Intermittent fasting is a very effective way to deal with when to eat. Essentially, the question is this:

If you don't eat, will you lose weight? Yes, of course you will. In this cookbook, I provide more than 100 recipes offering wonderful choices for when you do eat and delicious beverages for when you fast.

PRACTICAL FASTING FACTS AND FAQS

AS A HEALING tradition, fasting has long met with success. For example, among the treatments prescribed and championed by Hippocrates of Kos (c. 460–c. 370 BC), who is widely considered the father of modern medicine, were the practice of fasting and the consumption of apple cider vinegar. He wrote, "To eat when you are sick, is to feed your illness." Consider the last time you had the flu. Probably the last thing you wanted to do was eat.

Though fasting seems to be an instinctual and universal human response to multiple forms of illness, many people regard it with skepticism. Many fasting myths have been repeated so often they are accepted as truths.

Consider the following popular beliefs:
· Fasting will make you lose muscle/burn protein.
· The brain needs glucose to function.
· Fasting puts you in starvation mode/lowers basal metabolism.
· Fasting will overwhelm you with hunger.
· Fasting deprives the body of nutrients.
· Fasting causes hypoglycemia.

If these myths were true, none of us would be alive today. Think about the consequences of burning muscle for energy, for example. In prehistoric times, the long winters contained many days when no food was available. After the first cold snap resulting in food scarcity, if your body was burning muscle for energy, you would be severely weakened. After several instances, you would be so weak that you couldn't hunt or gather food. Our bodies do not burn muscle in the absence of food unless our body fat drops to below 4 percent. The average North American carries an estimated 25 to 30 percent body fat.

The truth is that fasting is just as effective at treating our modern illnesses—obesity, diabetes, the entire constellation of ailments resulting from metabolic syndrome—as those of our ancestors. Remember, fasting is *voluntarily* withholding food for a specific period of time. As with any major lifestyle change, consult with your physician before you begin—especially if you are pregnant or have diabetes. The following section provides more information about what fasting is and what to expect.

The Basics of Fasting

For the fasts I recommend, non-caloric drinks such as black coffee, clear broth, water, and tea are permitted to help suppress appetite and prevent dehydration. Fasting has no standard duration or interval; fasts can range from twelve hours to three months or more, with weekly, monthly, or annual intervals between them. Intermittent fasting involves fasting for shorter periods on a regular, more frequent basis. The three most common fasting periods I recommend are sixteen hours, twenty-four hours, and thirty-six hours.

- A daily sixteen-hour fast means you eat your meals within an eight-hour window. So, if you begin your fast at 7:00 p.m., for example, you don't eat anything until 11:00 a.m. the following day. You consume two or three meals from that point on and resume your fast at 7:00 p.m. that evening.

- For a twenty-four-hour fast, you fast from, for example, dinner at 7:00 p.m. on the first day until dinner at 7:00 p.m. the next day.

- For a thirty-six-hour fast, you fast from, for example, dinner at 7:00 p.m. on the first day until breakfast at 7:00 a.m. two days later.

Longer fasting periods produce lower insulin levels, greater weight loss, and greater blood sugar reduction in people with diabetes. In the clinic, I typically recommend a twenty-four-hour or thirty-six-hour fast, two or three times per week.

Ready to give it a try but still have some questions? Here are answers to some of the most common ones.

Fasting FAQS

WHAT CAN I CONSUME ON FASTING DAYS?

All calorie-containing foods and beverages are withheld during fasting. However, you must stay well hydrated throughout your fast. Water—still or sparkling—is always a good choice. Aim to drink eight cups (two liters) of water daily. You may add a squeeze of lemon or lime for flavor. Try diluted apple cider vinegar (simply dilute according to taste), which may help with your blood sugars. Homemade bone broth (pages 186–192), made from beef, pork, chicken, or fish bones and a good pinch of salt, is also a good choice for fasting days. Vegetable broth is a suitable alternative, although bone broth contains more nutrients. Avoid canned broths and bouillon cubes, which are full of artificial flavors and monosodium glutamate. Any form of sugar, artificial flavors, or sweeteners is prohibited during a fast.

I TAKE MEDICATIONS WITH FOOD. WHAT CAN I DO WHILE FASTING?

Certain medications may cause problems on an empty stomach. For example, Aspirin can cause stomach upset or even ulcers. Iron supplements may cause nausea and vomiting. Metformin, which is used to treat diabetes and polycystic ovary syndrome (PCOS), may cause nausea or diarrhea. Always discuss your medications with your physician before starting a fast.

I AM DIABETIC. CAN I FAST?

Special care must be taken if you have diabetes or you are taking diabetic medications, because fasting reduces blood sugars. If you are taking diabetic medications, especially insulin, your blood sugars may become extremely low, which can be a life-threatening situation. *Close medical monitoring by your physician is mandatory. If you cannot be followed closely, do not fast.*

In the Intensive Dietary Management program, I often reduce diabetes medications for patients before they start a fast in anticipation of lower blood sugars. However, since blood sugar response is unpredictable, check your blood sugars at least twice a day while fasting and record the information. If you have repeated low blood sugar results, you may be overmedicated. If your blood sugars become extremely low, though, you must take some sugar or juice to bring your sugars back to normal, even if it means you must stop your fast for that day. You should also check your blood pressure regularly, preferably weekly. Be sure to discuss routine blood work, including electrolyte measurement, with your physician. Should you feel unwell for any reason, stop your fast immediately and seek medical advice.

WHAT CAN I DO IF I GET HUNGRY WHILE FASTING?

This is probably the number one concern of fasters everywhere. People assume they'll be overwhelmed with hunger and unable to control themselves. The truth is that hunger does not persist; it comes in waves. If you're experiencing hunger, it will pass. Staying busy during a fasting day can help you resist the desire to eat. As the body becomes accustomed to fasting, it starts to burn its stores of fat, and your hunger will decrease. During longer fasts, many people notice that their hunger completely has disappeared by the second or third day.

CAN I EXERCISE WHILE FASTING?

Absolutely. There is no reason to stop your exercise routine. All types of exercise, including resistance (weights) and cardio, are encouraged. There is a common misperception that eating is necessary to supply "energy" to the working body. That's not true. The liver supplies energy via gluconeogenesis. During longer fasting periods, muscles use fatty acids directly for energy. In fact, because your adrenalin levels will be higher during fasting, it is an *ideal* time to exercise. The rise in growth hormone that comes with fasting may also promote muscle growth.

WILL FASTING MAKE ME TIRED?

Probably not. In my experience at the Intensive Dietary Management Clinic, the opposite is true. Many people find they have more energy during a fast—probably due to increased adrenalin levels. Basal metabolism does not fall during fasting; it rises. You'll find you can perform all the normal activities of daily living while fasting. Persistent or excessive fatigue is not a normal part of fasting. If you experience that, you should stop fasting immediately and seek medical advice.

WILL FASTING MAKE ME CONFUSED OR FORGETFUL?

You should not experience any decrease in memory or concentration during your fast. The ancient Greeks believed that fasting significantly improved cognitive abilities, helping the great thinkers attain more clarity and mental acuity. Over the long term, fasting may improve memory. One theory is that fasting activates a form of cellular cleansing called autophagy that may help prevent age-associated memory loss.

IF I GET DIZZY, WHAT CAN I DO?

If you're experiencing dizziness, you're most probably becoming dehydrated. Be sure to drink plenty of fluids and add extra salt to your broth or mineral water to help retain the fluids longer. Another possibility is that your blood pressure is too low, particularly if you're taking medications for hypertension. Speak to your physician about adjusting your medications. Persistent dizziness, nausea, or vomiting are not normal with intermittent or continuous fasting. If you experience any of these symptoms persistently, you should stop fasting immediately and seek medical advice.

IF I GET MUSCLE CRAMPS, WHAT CAN I DO?

Low magnesium levels, which are particularly common in people with diabetes, may cause muscle cramps. To address this, you may take an over-the-counter magnesium supplement or soak in Epsom salts, which are magnesium salts. Add one cup (250 milliliters) to a warm bath and soak in it for half an hour. The magnesium will be absorbed through your skin.

IF I GET A HEADACHE, WHAT CAN I DO?

Try increasing your salt intake by adding an extra pinch or two to your bone broth or mineral water. Headaches are quite common the first few times you try a fast. It is believed that they're caused by the transition from a relatively high-salt diet to very low salt intake on fasting days. They are usually temporary, and as you become accustomed to fasting, this problem often resolves itself. If you have any concerns about your headaches, speak to a physician.

IF I EXPERIENCE CONSTIPATION, WHAT CAN I DO?

It is not uncommon to experience constipation at the start of a fast. Increasing your intake of fiber, fruits, and vegetables during the non-fasting period may help. Metamucil can also be taken to increase fiber and stool bulk. If the problem continues, ask your doctor to consider prescribing a laxative.

HOW SHOULD I BREAK MY FAST?

Be careful to break your fast gently by starting with a handful of nuts or a small salad. Overeating right after fasting may lead to stomach discomfort or heartburn. While not serious, these conditions can be quite uncomfortable. Avoid lying down immediately after a meal; instead, try to stay upright for at least half an hour. If you experience heartburn at night, placing wooden blocks under the head of your bed to raise it may help. If none of these solutions work for you, consult your physician.

I'M NOT LOSING WEIGHT. WHAT'S WRONG?

If one of the goals of your fast is to lose weight, persist and be patient. The amount of weight loss varies tremendously from person to person. The longer you have struggled with obesity, the more difficult you'll find it to lose weight. Certain medications may make it hard to lose weight. And you'll probably eventually experience a weight-loss plateau. Changing your fasting or dietary regimen, or both, may help. Some patients fast for longer, going from a twenty-four-hour fast to a thirty-six- or even forty-eight-hour fasting period. Some people try eating only once a day, every day. Others try a continuous fast for an entire week. Changing the fasting protocol is often what's required to break through a plateau, but consult with your physician to determine what might be right for you.

Tips for Success

At the Intensive Dietary Management Clinic, we help hundreds of people of all ages and with varying health conditions fast successfully every year. Here are some tips that may help you.

1. **Drink water**: Start each morning with a glass of water.

2. **Stay busy**: It'll keep your mind off food. It helps to choose a busy day at work when you're planning to fast.

3. **Drink coffee**: Coffee is a mild appetite suppressant. Also try green tea, black tea, and bone broth.

4. **Ride the waves**: Hunger comes in waves; it is not continuous. Be patient and distract yourself.

5. **Don't tell everybody you're fasting**: People may try to discourage you if they don't understand the benefits.

6. **Give yourself thirty days**: It takes time for your body to get used to fasting. Don't be discouraged if you experience a setback. It will get easier.

7. **Follow a nutritious diet on non-fasting days**: Intermittent fasting is not an excuse to eat whatever you like on non-fasting days. Stick to a nutritious diet that is low in sugars and refined carbohydrates.

8. **Don't binge**: After a fast, pretend it never happened. Eat normally, as if you had never fasted.

The last and most important tip is to fit fasting into your life! Arrange your fasting schedule so that it works with your lifestyle and do not limit yourself socially because you're fasting. There will be times during which it's impossible to fast: vacations, holidays, weddings, for example. Do not try to force fasting into these celebrations. These occasions are times to relax and enjoy yourself. Afterward, just resume your regular fasting schedule. While changing your diet may seem daunting, know that by making the decision to do so you've already taken the first step to better health.

RECIPES

Pantry

═══════════

THE RECIPES IN this book emphasize natural healthy fats and de-emphasize starches and sugars. You'll find assertive flavors in dishes prepared using easy techniques, and an overall philosophy that is permissive and flexible, not dogmatic. As you grow familiar with the recipe blueprints, feel free to substitute ingredients, adjust quantities, and lengthen or shorten cooking times according to your preferences.

Your experiments will be much easier if you have a good selection of basics in your pantry. It's particularly important that you read the labels of any commercially prepared sauces, condiments, dips, soups, and even spice blends before you buy or consume them. Sugar in its many forms is often added to prepared foods as an inexpensive flavoring and various highly refined starches are added as thickeners.

Here are some pantry staples to keep on hand.

Beverages

In this cookbook, I provide many ideas for beverages allowed during fasts, including bone broths. Here are a few options so that you're never bored with your drinks.

- Coffee: caffeinated and decaffeinated
- Tea: black, white, green, oolong, herbal, Pique tea crystals (piquetea. com)
- Water: obviously! Still or sparkling, filtered or tap; try flavoring with tea crystals
- Dry red wine: in moderation during non-fasting periods; confirm low sugar content

Condiments

Commercial condiments are very often loaded with added sugars. Be on the lookout for any ingredients ending in "-ose," as they are often sugars in disguise. Become a regular label reader! Here are the real utility players:

- Curry paste
- Dijon and grainy mustard
- Miso (soybean paste)
- Sambal oelek (chili paste)
- Tahini (sesame paste)
- Tamari (gluten-free soy sauce)

Dairy

Choose full-fat, full-flavor options when it comes to dairy. Use butter, cheese, and cream to thicken and fortify sauces or finish dishes. If cow's milk doesn't suit you, try goat's or sheep's milk. Avoid margarines. Keep the following in your fridge:

- Butter (salted or unsalted, whichever you prefer), full-fat milk, 18% and 35% cream
- Cheese, hard, soft and semi-soft, ricotta: you won't go wrong if you always have some Parmesan or Pecorino to hand
- Yogurt: avoid sweetened varieties with added fruit

Oils

Avoid oils that are overly refined or processed. This includes many vegetable oils, such as corn, safflower, cottonseed, and canola oil. Instead, choose cold-pressed oils as close to the original food source as possible.

- Coconut oil
- Extra virgin olive oil
- Ghee (clarified butter)
- Grapeseed oil
- Toasted sesame oil
- Walnut oil

Protein

Moderate your intake of protein. You don't need huge amounts to feel satisfied and energetic, but do try to eat some protein with every meal.

- Beans: dried and canned, a good way to add fiber to your diet
- Eggs: a great choice; don't just save them for breakfast
- Fish, poultry, red and white meats: opt for fattier choices and always have bacon, prosciutto, or pancetta handy; they freeze well
- Nuts and seeds: walnuts, almonds, sesame seeds, flax seeds, sunflower seeds, chia seeds
- Quinoa: remember this isn't a grain, it's a seed

Spices

Dried spices and herbs lose their flavor more rapidly than most people realize. It's better to have fewer spices in circulation and use them within three months, if possible.

- Black pepper
- Chili flakes and chili powder
- Chipotle pepper
- Cumin, ground and seeds

- Curry powder
- Herbes de Provence (dried basil, oregano, lavender, rosemary, fennel, thyme, tarragon)
- Ground turmeric

Sweeteners

If you choose to have honey or maple syrup in your pantry, be certain that it doesn't contain any high-fructose corn syrup. Choose pure maple syrup and be sure to avoid products labeled as "pancake syrup."

Vegetables and Fruits

Eat your veggies! It's simple. Try adding some healthy fats for a little extra flavor—olive oil will do the trick. Avoid white potatoes if you're trying to lose weight. Opt for fresh or frozen vegetables; canned aren't the best choice, although you should have canned tomatoes on hand at all times—they're not only flavorful, they're also very versatile.

- Canned tomatoes
- Citrus: lemons and limes add bright flavor and acidity
- Ginger root: it freezes, making it easier to grate
- Leafy, dark green vegetables, such as kale, chard, collards, and broccoli
- Olives packed in olive oil
- Onions, green onions, shallots, garlic: always have a selection of the allium family on hand

Vinegar

Fermented foods and liquids help with digestion. They also add an acidic brightness to counterbalance richness. Be careful with balsamic vinegar, which often has a high sugar content. This is particularly true of flavored balsamic vinegars. Other vinegars infused with herbs, such as tarragon, are wonderful in salad dressings, as is apple cider vinegar.

- Apple cider vinegar
- Red wine and white wine vinegar
- Rice wine vinegar
- Sherry vinegar

BREAK
THE FAST

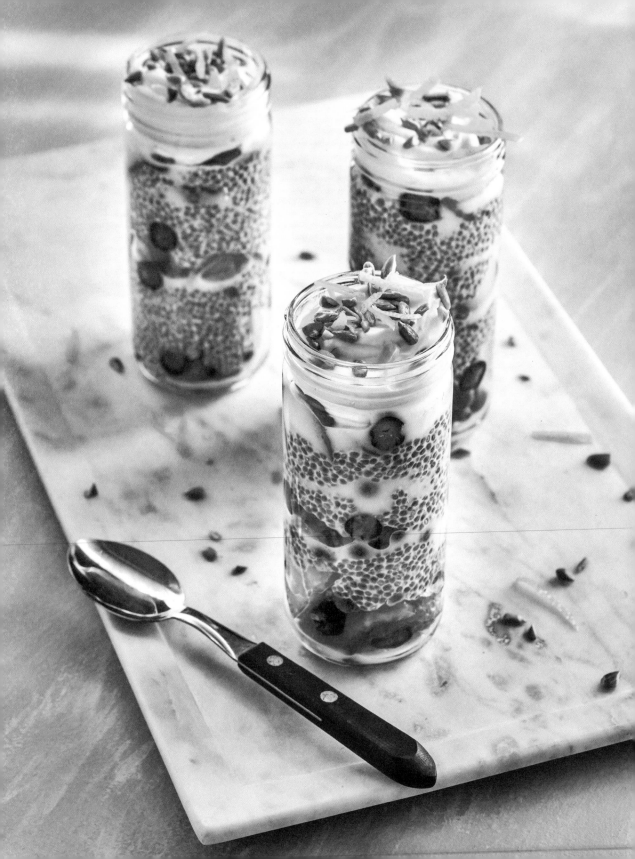

CHIA SEED PARFAITS

Adaptable and delicious, chia seed pudding is wildly popular for good reason. The seeds offer antioxidants, protein, and fiber. Almost all the carbohydrates in chia seeds are fiber, not starches or sugars, making them a great addition to a low-carbohydrate kitchen. When chia seeds are combined with liquid, they become gelatinous, with a pudding-like consistency that readily absorbs flavorings.

MAKES 4 SERVINGS

4 cups/1 L unsweetened coconut or almond milk

Pure vanilla extract or ground cinnamon to taste

Kosher salt

1 cup/250 mL chia seeds

2 cups/500 mL fresh or frozen berries

4 Tbsp/60 mL chopped nuts and seeds

Grated lemon zest, for garnish

1. Assemble and measure ingredients. Have ready four 12-ounce/350 milliliter glass jars with lids.

2. In a glass measuring cup, combine milk with vanilla (or cinnamon) and a pinch of salt. Whisk in chia seeds.

3. Divide a third of the berries among the jars followed by a third of the chia mixture. Repeat with two more layers of each. Top with a tablespoon of nuts and seeds and a sprinkle of lemon zest. Cover and refrigerate overnight or for up to 3 days.

4. Serve cold or at room temperature.

BERRIES WITH ROASTED NUTS AND CREAM

Make this with your favorite berries—or whichever ones look most luscious at the market. Same goes for the nuts. This dish makes a lovely breakfast or dessert with a healthy dose of fiber, fat, and protein. A little maple syrup provides sweetness and makes it more of a treat than an everyday dish.

MAKES 4 SERVINGS

1 lb/450 g mixed fresh berries

1 lb/450 g mixed raw nuts

2 sprigs fresh rosemary

2 Tbsp butter

½ tsp cayenne pepper (optional)

1 tsp pure maple syrup or granulated maple syrup (optional)

Salt flakes or coarse crystals

1 cup/250 mL 18% or 35% cream or Greek yogurt

1. Assemble, prepare, and measure ingredients. Rinse and drain berries well. Spread them out on a clean tea towel for a few minutes to dry them off completely, then move to a wide, shallow bowl. Chop nuts roughly into large pieces. Pick rosemary leaves and mince very finely. Preheat oven to 350°F/180°C.

2. Melt butter in a large straight-sided skillet over medium heat. Add cayenne and/or maple syrup (if using). Stir in nuts to coat well and then toast for 2–3 minutes. Move nuts to an ungreased baking sheet, sprinkle with salt and rosemary, and bake for 10–15 minutes, or until nuts are deep brown in places and your kitchen smells wonderful. Remove nuts from oven and allow to cool and crisp up before using.

3. To serve, divide berries among four bowls. Pour some cream or spoon some yogurt over berries and top with a couple of tablespoons of toasted nuts. If you choose to use 35% cream, you can whip it but don't add sugar.

EASY EVERYDAY OMELET

An omelet is a classic and satisfying way to eat eggs that also provides
an elegant solution if you're feeding picky eaters: just vary the fillings
according to people's preferences. I always like to include cheese in my omelet
filling because it melts so well in the heat of the eggy envelope.

MAKES 4 SERVINGS

8 eggs

Olive oil, to sauté filling

⅓ cup/80 mL omelet filling
    per person (see note)

8 tsp butter

Salt and pepper

1. Assemble, prepare, and measure ingredients. Beat eggs with
   ¼ cup/60mL water, and salt and pepper. Sauté ingredients
   for omelet filling, if necessary.

2. Melt 2 teaspoons butter in a small nonstick sauté pan over
   medium-high heat. Slowly pour in a quarter of the beaten
   eggs and tilt pan until they completely cover the surface.
   Use a wooden spoon to move any uncooked egg from the
   edges to the center, and cook until omelet has set around
   the edges but middle is still runny.

3. Sprinkle filling down the center of the omelet. Use a spatula to fold one-third of the omelet toward the middle. Hold
   the pan over a plate and gently roll the omelet out of the
   pan, folding the other edge into the middle as you do so.

4. Repeat to make three more filled omelets. Serve
   immediately.

Note: Classic fillings for omelets include cheeses, cooked meats or seafood, and sautéed vegetables, but
don't be afraid to raid your fridge to use up leftovers. Here are some filling ideas to get you started:
- Brie & ham: cut cheese and ham into small cubes
- Cheddar & sautéed shallots: cut cheese into small cubes, sauté one large or two small shallots for 5
  minutes in a drizzle of olive oil
- Mozzarella & arugula: cut cheese into small cubes, tear arugula leaves roughly

COCONUT PANCAKES

These pancakes are a wonderful treat. Coconut flour is higher in fiber
than wheat flour, so it's a better choice for your digestion and blood sugar levels.
To make these extra delicious, top each serving with a mixture of berries and
a spoonful of heavy cream. They're also great with bacon—but isn't everything?

MAKES 4 SERVINGS

2 Tbsp coconut oil or butter,
plus more for cooking

6 eggs

1 cup/250 mL coconut milk or
cow's milk

1 tsp pure vanilla extract

½ cup/125 mL coconut flour

1 tsp baking soda

Salt

1. Assemble, prepare, and measure ingredients. Melt coconut oil (or butter) and cool to room temperature. Whisk eggs vigorously until fully combined.

2. In a mixing bowl, stir melted coconut oil (or butter), milk, and vanilla into beaten eggs. Sift in flour and baking soda. Add a pinch of salt. If batter seems too thick, add some more milk, about 1 tablespoon at a time.

3. Heat a griddle or frying pan over medium-high heat until a droplet of water hisses and dances on the surface. Heat about 1 teaspoon coconut oil or butter in the pan. Ladle in three little pancakes, each no larger than 3 inches/7.5 cm in diameter or they will break when you flip them.

4. Watch them closely. They will brown and start to smell ready after 2–3 minutes. Flip them carefully and cook for another 2 minutes.

5. Serve right away, preferably with berries and cream over top.

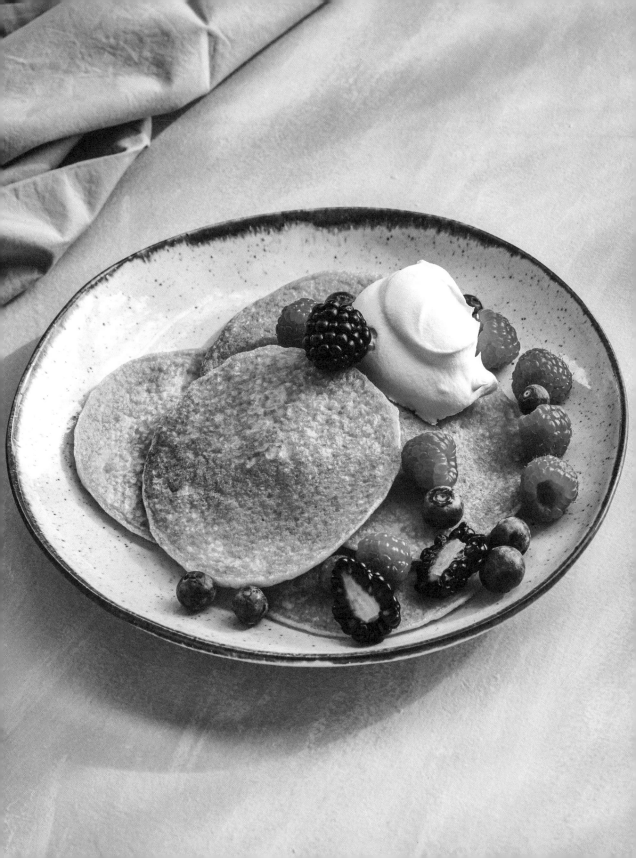

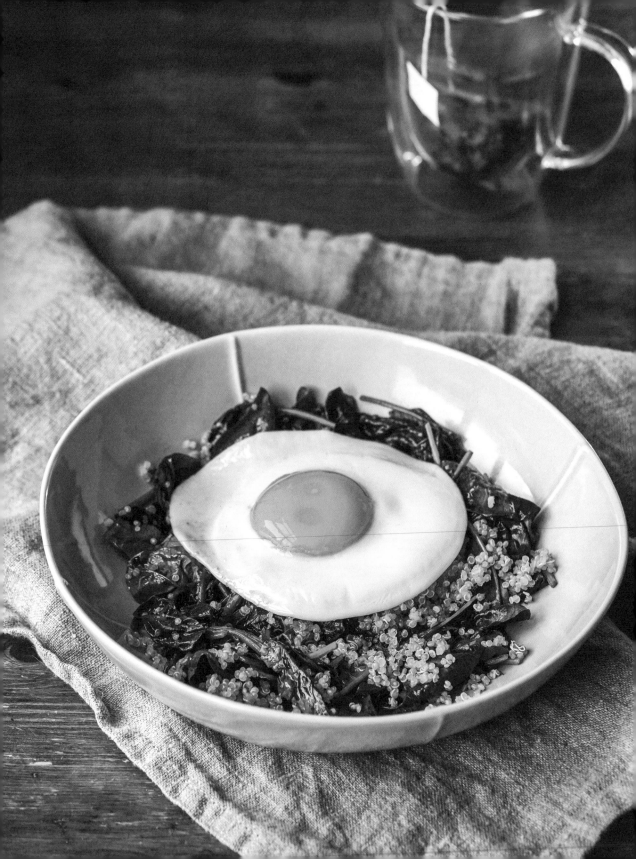

FRIED EGGS WITH
SPICY SPINACH AND QUINOA

For those of you who love to have breakfast for dinner, this dish has it all:
it's rich and spicy, with bright green flavors. Plenty of protein from the powerhouse
eggs and quinoa gives you the staying power to get out there and get things
done! Serve with extra harissa or your favorite hot sauce on the side.

MAKES 4 SERVINGS

½ cup/125 mL quinoa

2 Tbsp butter

2 Tbsp olive oil

4 eggs

½ lb/225 g spinach

1 tsp harissa paste or chili
 flakes

Salt and pepper

1. Assemble and measure ingredients.

2. Bring 1 cup/250 mL salted water to a boil in a small saucepan. Add quinoa, cover, turn down heat to low, and cook for
   15–20 minutes, or until quinoa forms little "tails." Remove
   from heat. If there is any remaining water, drain quinoa in a
   fine-mesh sieve. Set aside in saucepan or sieve, uncovered.

3. Heat two heavy-bottomed skillets over medium heat. Melt
   1 tablespoon of butter with 1 tablespoon of olive oil in each
   skillet.

4. Turn down heat to low under one skillet. Crack eggs into it
   and cook very slowly, until whites are opaque and yolks are
   still runny, about 5 minutes.

5. Meanwhile, add several handfuls of spinach to the other
   skillet and allow to wilt. Add remaining spinach, handful by
   handful, as space allows. When spinach has all wilted, stir in
   harissa paste (or chili flakes). Season with salt and pepper.

6. To serve, divide spicy spinach among four bowls, spoon
   quinoa over top, and top with a fried egg. Drizzle pan juices
   over top and serve.

SAVORY GRUYERE CUSTARD

Another egg dish that could be served at any time of day, this cheesy custard would be perfectly balanced by a green salad with a lemon vinaigrette. Frisée, mâche, Boston, or butter lettuce with Simple Vinaigrette (page 80) would do the trick.

MAKES 4 SERVINGS

2 oz/55 g Gruyere cheese

2 oz/55 g Parmesan or
   Pecorino cheese

2 cups/500 mL 35% cream

1 sprig fresh thyme

1 garlic clove

3 eggs

3 egg yolks

½ tsp dry mustard or ground
   cayenne

Salt and pepper

1. Assemble, prepare, and measure ingredients. Grate both cheeses. Preheat oven to 300°F/150°C. Lightly butter four 1-cup/250 mL ramekins or a 1-quart/1 L baking dish.

2. In a small saucepan, warm cream over medium-low heat with thyme and garlic until steam rises. Remove from heat and allow to infuse and cool while you make the eggs.

3. In a mixing bowl, beat eggs and yolks with mustard (or cayenne) and salt and pepper. Stir in grated cheeses. Strain cream through a fine-mesh sieve and whisk into egg mixture.

4. Pour custard mixture into ramekins (or baking dish) and place in a large roasting pan. Pour boiling water around dishes to come halfway up their sides. Be careful not to splash any water into the custards, as you want them to be creamy and silken, not watery. Bake for 30–45 minutes, or until center is just set. Custards in ramekins will cook more quickly than those in a single baking dish. Remove from oven and allow to cool slightly.

5. To serve, place ramekins on individual plates or scoop out individual servings from larger baking dish.

SCRAMBLED EGGS WITH SMOKED SALMON AND DILL

Despite what you may have read, there is no need to overthink your technique when making scrambled eggs. They can be whipped up quickly; life is too short to measure the size of the curds. And feel free to adapt this classic recipe to your preferences (or the ingredients in your fridge): in place of smoked salmon and dill, try one or both variations below (see note) or invent your own version. Cleanup is easier when you cook eggs on a nonstick surface, but there is enough butter in this recipe to avoid sticking.

MAKES 4 SERVINGS

8 eggs

4 oz/100 g smoked salmon

3 sprigs fresh dill

2 Tbsp butter

Salt and pepper

1. Assemble, prepare, and measure ingredients. Beat eggs with salt and pepper. Slice smoked salmon into ribbons. Using sharp scissors, snip dill fronds and discard stems.

2. In a medium skillet over medium-low heat, melt butter. Pour eggs into skillet and stir gently with a wooden spoon, moving cooked eggs to allow uncooked eggs to flow over skillet surface, for about 2 minutes, or until soft curds form. The eggs will still be runny. Remove skillet from heat.

3. Immediately fold smoked salmon and dill into the scrambled eggs and allow mixture to sit for another minute or so to finish cooking eggs.

4. Serve warm.

Note: Scrambled eggs are very versatile. Here are a couple of variations to get you started.
- Chèvre & chive: In step 2, cook eggs with 2 oz/55 g crumbled chèvre. In step 3, omit smoked salmon and fold in 3–5 minced fresh chives in place of dill.
- Mushrooms & thyme: In step 2, cook ½ lb/225 g sliced button mushrooms for 5 minutes until mushrooms release their liquid and it evaporates, then add eggs. In step 3, omit smoked salmon and fold in leaves from two sprigs of fresh thyme in place of dill.

POACHED EGGS ON SPINACH WITH PROSCIUTTO

The trickiest thing about this recipe is getting the poached eggs right. Adding vinegar to the simmering water is a traditional—but risky—way to help the whites to form. If you get the quantity of vinegar wrong, you get horrid, rubbery egg whites. Yuck. Instead, make a whirlpool! This method works and you'll feel like a pro.

MAKES 4 SERVINGS

4 eggs
2 garlic cloves
2–3 Tbsp olive oil
1 lb/450 g spinach
½ lb/225 g prosciutto slices
Salt and pepper

1. Assemble, prepare, and measure ingredients. Crack eggs into teacups or ramekins. Thinly slice garlic. Line a plate with paper towels.

2. Bring a small saucepan of water to a boil. Turn down heat, make a whirlpool with a wooden spoon, and gently slide in two eggs. Set a timer for 3 minutes. When eggs are poached, carefully remove them to the plate with a slotted spoon. Repeat with the other two eggs.

3. In a skillet large enough to hold all the spinach, warm olive oil over medium heat and stir in garlic. Sauté garlic very briefly, then toss spinach in by the handful, adding more as it wilts. Once spinach has all wilted, turn off heat. Season with salt and pepper, remove to a bowl, and keep warm.

4. In the same skillet, add some olive oil if necessary and quickly crisp prosciutto slices, about 30 seconds per side.

5. To serve, make a nest of spinach on each of four plates. Top with a poached egg, season with salt and pepper, and serve with a couple of prosciutto slices on the side.

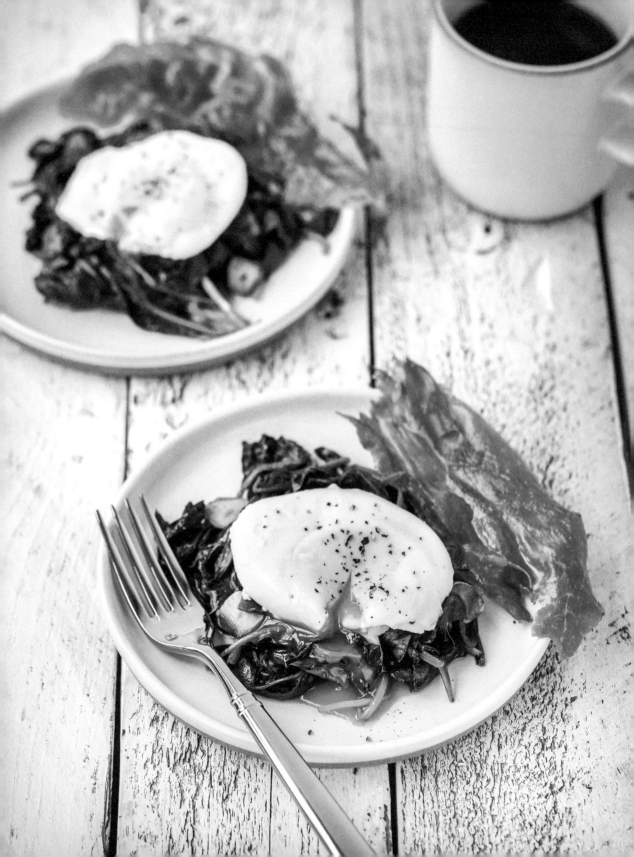

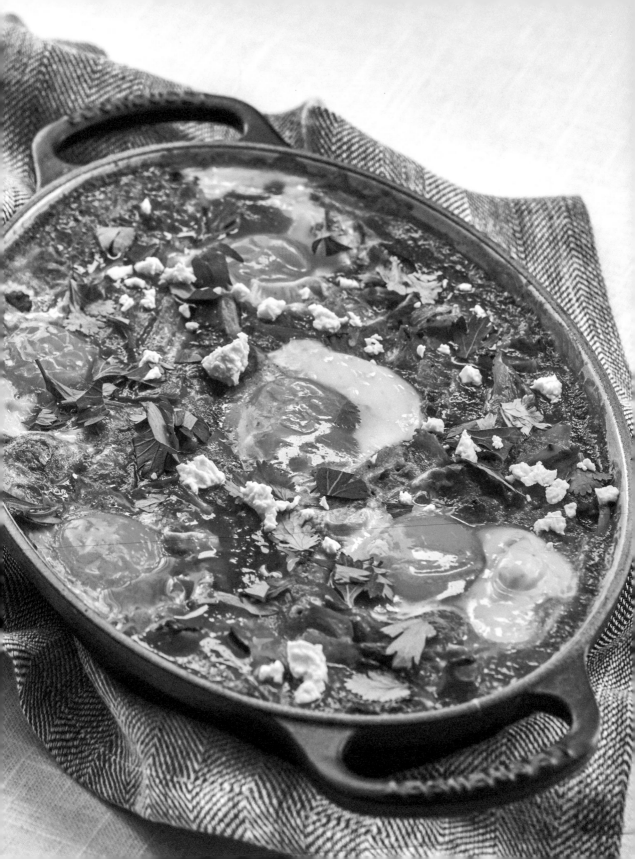

SHAKSHUKA

From the culinary traditions of Israel and North Africa, this thick, quick, spicy tomato sauce makes a perfect braise for eggs. It's an aromatic feast, good to eat at any time of day. The feta cheese provides enough fat to keep you feeling satisfied for hours.

MAKES 4 SERVINGS

2 yellow onions
2 red bell peppers
4 garlic cloves
3 Tbsp olive oil
1 tsp ground cumin
1 tsp cayenne pepper
2 Tbsp tomato paste
1 can (28 oz/796 mL) whole tomatoes (with juice reserved)
8 eggs
4 sprigs fresh cilantro
1 bunch flat-leaf parsley
3 oz/80 g creamy feta cheese
Salt and pepper

1. Assemble, prepare, and measure ingredients. Thinly slice onions. Chop bell peppers. Mince garlic.

2. In a wide straight-sided saucepan, heat olive oil over medium heat. Sauté onions and peppers for 5 minutes, or until soft. Add garlic and cook for 1 minute. Season with salt and pepper. Add cumin and cayenne, and stir in tomato paste. Cook for 2–3 minutes, or until tomato paste starts to caramelize. Add tomatoes with their juice. Season again with salt and pepper.

3. Simmer gently (just a few bubbles), uncovered, for 10–15 minutes to reduce liquid. The sauce should be thick enough to hold an indentation from the back of your spoon.

4. Make eight indentations in the sauce and carefully crack a whole egg into each one. (This is easiest to do if you crack each egg into a ramekin and pour it into the sauce.) Season with salt and pepper. Cover and cook for 3 minutes, or until whites are set and yolks are cooked to your liking.

5. Roughly tear cilantro and parsley and scatter over shakshuka. Crumble feta evenly over sauce, avoiding eggs.

6. To serve, divide shakshuka among four bowls, giving everyone two eggs.

SOFT-BOILED EGGS
WITH ROASTED ASPARAGUS

If you're not in the habit of eating boiled eggs, you may not have any
egg cups handy. If so, here's a good serving trick: nestle the eggs into a bed of raw
rice or coarse salt in a teacup or small ramekin. The eggs will remain upright
and you will have some room to maneuver as you cut off the tops with a very sharp
knife. Asparagus spears make a perfect stand-in for toast fingers.

MAKES 4 SERVINGS

1 lb/450 g asparagus spears
1 Tbsp olive oil
4 eggs
Salt and pepper

1. Assemble, prepare, and measure ingredients. Snap tough, woody ends off asparagus. Preheat oven to 400°F/200°C.

2. Spread asparagus in a single layer on an unlined, ungreased baking sheet. Drizzle with olive oil. Season with salt and pepper. Roast for 15–18 minutes, or until dark brown in places.

3. Meanwhile, bring a medium saucepan of water to a vigorous boil. Turn down heat to get a rapid simmer (many small bubbles) and, using a spoon, gently lower eggs into water. Cook eggs for 5 minutes and then remove from water.

4. To serve, set soft-boiled eggs in egg cups and cut off tops. Arrange roasted asparagus on a serving plate and invite your guests to use them for dipping into warm yolks. Use a small spoon to eat cooked whites.

SIGNIFICANT
SALADS

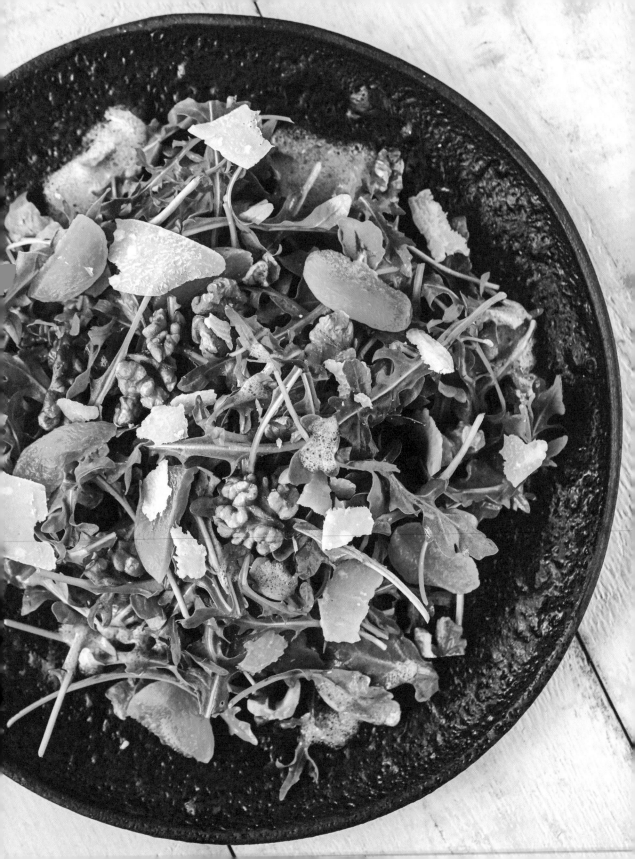

ARUGULA, FIG, AND WALNUT SALAD WITH BACON VINAIGRETTE

Many culinary traditions add bacon—or bacon bits, pancetta, or lardons—to salads. Why not use some of the delicious fat in a salad dressing? It adds depth and a hit of salt to complement the nuts and greens in this deceptively simple entrée.

MAKES 4 SERVINGS

SALAD

4 fresh figs or 8 dried prunes or apricots
3 oz/80 g Parmesan cheese
½ cup/70 g walnut halves or pieces
3 slices bacon
8 cups/160 g arugula

BACON VINAIGRETTE

2 Tbsp rendered bacon fat
6 Tbsp olive oil
2 Tbsp white wine vinegar
1 Tbsp Dijon mustard
Salt and pepper

1. Assemble, prepare, and measure ingredients. Quarter figs lengthwise (or halve prunes or dried apricots lengthwise). Using a vegetable peeler or cheese pull, shave Parmesan.

2. Place walnut pieces in an ungreased skillet and toast over medium-low heat for about 5 minutes, or until they release their nutty scent. Let cool in the pan.

3. Fry bacon in a separate skillet over low heat for 15 minutes, or until fat has rendered. Drain off and reserve fat. Dry and blot bacon with paper towel. Crumble bacon when it's cool enough to handle.

4. For the vinaigrette, in a small bowl, combine 2 tablespoons of reserved bacon fat with olive oil, vinegar, mustard, and salt and pepper. Whisk to emulsify, adding more olive oil or vinegar, 1 teaspoon at a time, if necessary. Taste and adjust seasoning, if necessary.

5. For the salad, tip arugula into a large salad bowl. Add vinaigrette and toss gently but thoroughly. Distribute figs (or prunes or dried apricots), Parmesan, walnuts, and bacon evenly over top. Don't toss salad again or the small pieces will sink to the bottom of the bowl. Serve soon after dressing salad.

ASPARAGUS MIMOSA WITH CHAMPAGNE VINAIGRETTE

Food and drink puns galore! A mimosa is a lovely white and yellow flower, the colors of the grated hard-boiled egg sprinkled over the vivid green asparagus in a mimosa salad. It's also a classic brunch cocktail, represented here by the champagne and orange juice vinaigrette. Scrumptious food for thought.

MAKES 4 SERVINGS

2 bunches asparagus

6 chives

2 large eggs

1 Tbsp champagne vinegar

½ cup/125 mL olive oil

2 Tbsp fresh orange juice

Salt and pepper

1. Assemble, prepare, and measure ingredients. Snap tough, woody ends off asparagus. Mince chives.

2. In a small saucepan, cover eggs with cold water and bring to a boil. Immediately remove eggs from heat and let sit in hot water for 12 minutes.

3. Meanwhile, place asparagus in a saucepan, cover with cold water, and bring to a boil over high heat. Let boil, uncovered, for 5 minutes, then drain and dry well on a clean tea towel.

4. Drain eggs and gently roll on a countertop to crack shells. Peel under cold running water and set aside.

5. In a small bowl, whisk vinegar with olive oil and orange juice. Season with salt and pepper.

6. Arrange asparagus on a serving platter. Drizzle with champagne vinaigrette. Working directly over asparagus, push hard-boiled eggs through a fine-mesh sieve or use a microplane grater to grate them. Season with salt and pepper. Scatter chives over top and serve.

CAPRESE SALAD

The key to this salad is the interplay of fresh mozzarella, perfectly ripe tomatoes, basil, and the best olive oil you can afford. Feel free to use little grape tomatoes and bocconcini, or gorgeous heirloom tomatoes and torn burrata. This is also a perfect time to use salt flakes and coarsely ground peppercorns, if you have them. And you can make a quick pesto dressing of garlic, basil, pine nuts, and olive oil to drizzle over the cheese and tomatoes if you want more intense flavor.

MAKES 4 SERVINGS

4 large, ripe tomatoes
½ lb/225 g fresh buffalo
   mozzarella
1 bunch fresh basil
¼ cup/60 mL olive oil
Salt and pepper

1. Assemble, prepare, and measure ingredients. Core and slice tomatoes, place on a platter, sprinkle lightly with salt, and set aside. Tear mozzarella into rough chunks. Pick basil leaves from stalks and roughly chop.

2. Drain juices from tomatoes by gently tilting the platter. Arrange tomatoes on platter—no need to rinse it—and distribute mozzarella and then basil evenly over top. Drizzle with olive oil. Season with salt and pepper. Serve.

BURRATA, ASPARAGUS, AND RADISH SALAD WITH LIME VINAIGRETTE

If you have never eaten burrata, you are in for a life-changing treat. It's mozzarella made with cow's milk or buffalo milk and cream. Imagine firm, chewy mozzarella on the outside and luscious creamy goodness on the inside. Now, try it with wafer-thin crunchy vegetables in a sprightly lime dressing. Perfect!

MAKES 4 SERVINGS

SALAD

1 bunch asparagus

12 radishes

1 English cucumber

½ lb/225 g burrata

LIME VINAIGRETTE

1 lime

6 Tbsp olive oil

1 Tbsp white wine vinegar

Salt and pepper

1. Assemble, prepare, and measure ingredients. Using a vegetable peeler or mandoline, shave asparagus spears into long, thin slices. Using a knife, slice radishes as thinly as possible. Using a knife, slice cucumber thinly. Tear the burrata into rough chunks. Zest and juice the lime.

2. For the salad, divide asparagus, radishes, and cucumber among four plates. Nestle burrata pieces among the vegetables.

3. For the vinaigrette, in a small bowl, whisk 1 teaspoon of lime zest with 1 tablespoon of lime juice, olive oil, and vinegar. Season with salt and pepper. Drizzle over salad and serve.

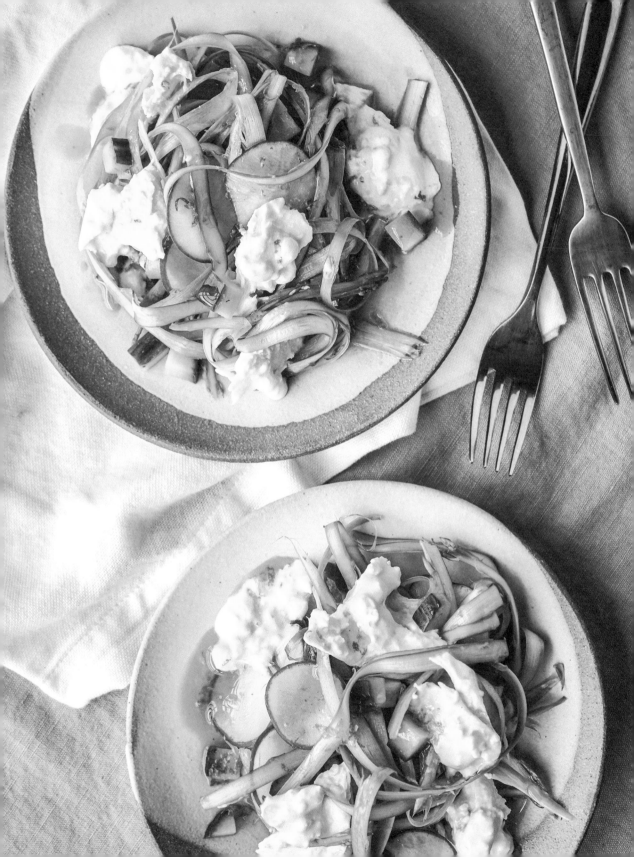

CHOPPED CHICKEN, AVOCADO, AND GRUYERE SALAD

A chopped salad fit for serving to guests or packing into containers to take for lunch. It's worth cooking the chicken just before serving because it's at its juicy best right out of the skillet. But the combination of creamy avocado, nutty Gruyere, and chicken is a flavorful protein hit no matter when you eat this.

MAKES 4 SERVINGS

SALAD

1 lb/450 g boneless, skinless chicken breasts

1 avocado

1 lb/450 g grape or cherry tomatoes

4 oz/100 g Gruyere cheese

2 Tbsp olive oil

2 tsp dried oregano

2 bunches arugula

Salt and pepper

DRESSING

1 lemon

1 garlic clove

¼ cup/60 mL olive oil

2 Tbsp mayonnaise

1 tsp Dijon mustard

1. Assemble, prepare, and measure ingredients. Cube chicken. Cut avocado in half, discard pit, scoop out and roughly chop flesh. Halve tomatoes. Grate Gruyere. Juice lemon. Mince garlic.

2. Warm 2 tablespoons of olive oil in a heavy-bottomed skillet over medium-high heat. Add chicken and season with oregano and salt and pepper. Sauté for 8–10 minutes, turning every so often to cook evenly. Remove from heat and allow to cool to room temperature in skillet.

3. For the dressing, in a small bowl, whisk 1 tablespoon of lemon juice with garlic, olive oil, mayonnaise, and mustard. Season with salt and pepper.

4. For the salad, arrange arugula on a large platter. Pour dressing over greens. Form separate piles of cooked chicken, avocado, and tomatoes atop arugula. Scatter Gruyere over everything and season well with salt and pepper. Serve.

RED AND SAVOY CABBAGE SLAW
WITH CRÈME FRAÎCHE

Cabbage is a cruciferous vegetable from the same family as broccoli, Brussels sprouts, and kale. Good for your fiber and nutrient intake, it's also the perfect crunchy vehicle for this sophisticated take on slaw dressing, with crème fraîche instead of commercially prepared mayo. If you can't find crème fraîche, use full-fat sour cream.

MAKES 4 SERVINGS

½ lb/225 g red cabbage

½ lb/225 g Savoy cabbage

3 carrots

1 green onion

½ cup/125 mL crème fraîche

2 Tbsp olive oil

2 Tbsp apple cider vinegar

1 tsp celery seed

Salt and pepper

1. Assemble, prepare, and measure ingredients. Using a knife, mandoline, or food processor, very finely slice or shred both cabbages. Using a box grater or mandoline, shred carrots. Mince white part of green onion.

2. Toss vegetables in a large nonreactive bowl.

3. In a small bowl, whisk crème fraîche with olive oil, vinegar, and celery seed. Season with salt and pepper. Pour dressing over shredded vegetables and toss well to coat thoroughly.

4. Cover and refrigerate for at least an hour before serving, if possible.

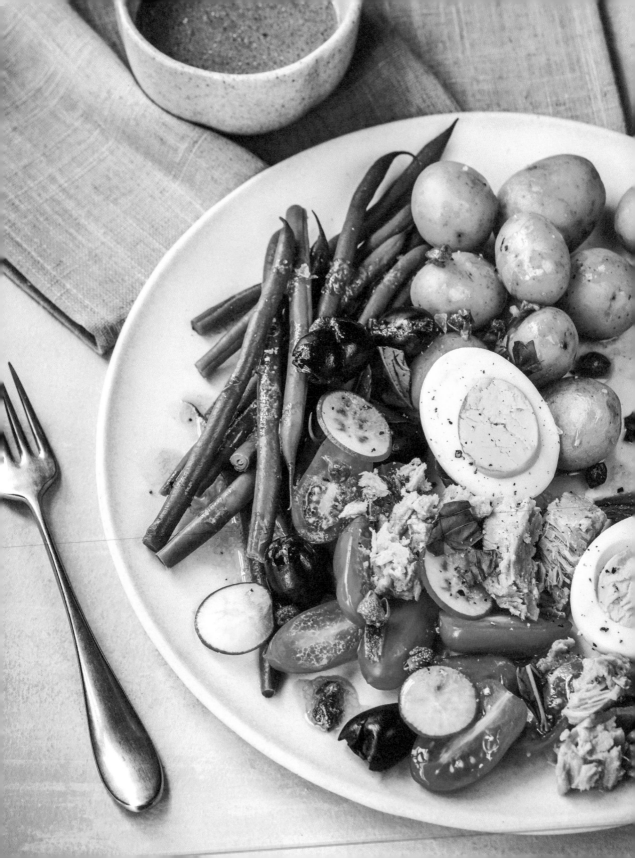

NIÇOISE SALAD

Some chefs say that a true salade Niçoise doesn't contain potatoes. You may certainly omit them if you want to adhere to tradition… or if you are trying to lose weight. New potatoes are less starchy than their adult relatives, but they are easily replaced by radishes and green beans, if you prefer.

MAKES 4 SERVINGS

SALAD

1 lb/450 g slender green
    beans
1 lb/450 g grape tomatoes
½ lb/225 g radishes
Handful basil leaves
1 lb/450 g new potatoes
4 eggs
1 cup/150 g black olives
12 anchovies
2 Tbsp capers
1 lb/450 g tuna packed in
    olive oil
Salt and pepper

DIJON VINAIGRETTE

2 Tbsp white wine vinegar
2 tsp Dijon mustard
6 Tbsp olive oil
Salt and pepper

1. Assemble, prepare, and measure ingredients. Trim beans. Halve tomatoes. Thinly slice radishes. Tear basil leaves roughly.

2. Place potatoes in a saucepan, cover with water, add 1 tablespoon salt, and bring to a boil over high heat. Boil for 12–15 minutes, or until fork-tender.

3. In a small saucepan, cover eggs with cold water and bring to a boil over high heat. Boil for about 5 minutes. Immediately remove eggs from heat, drain, and gently roll on countertop to crack shells. Peel eggs under cold running water and set aside.

4. Fill a large bowl with ice water. Bring a small saucepan of salted water to a boil, add beans, and blanch for about 4 minutes. Plunge into ice water to stop cooking, then drain.

5. For the vinaigrette, in a small bowl, whisk together vinegar and mustard. Slowly add olive oil, whisking to emulsify. Season with salt and pepper.

6. For the salad, arrange green beans, tomatoes, radishes, potatoes, olives, anchovies, and capers on each plate. Drizzle with some dressing. Add halved hard-boiled eggs and tuna to each plate. Scatter basil leaves over top and season with salt and pepper. Serve with extra dressing on the side.

ROASTED AND RAW SALADS: MUSHROOM AND FENNEL, BEET AND CARROT

Roasting vegetables adds a depth of flavor that combines well with raw greens to make a very satisfying salad. Use any firm vegetables that will hold their shape after roasting. Try green beans, parsnips, sweet potatoes, or white turnips. Get creative with herbs and spices and you'll never have the same salad twice.

MAKES 4 SERVINGS

SIMPLE VINAIGRETTE

1 lemon

1 Tbsp olive oil

1 tsp Dijon mustard

Salt and pepper

1. Assemble, prepare, and measure ingredients. Juice lemon.

2. In a small bowl, whisk together 2 tablespoons of lemon juice with olive oil and mustard. Season with salt and pepper. Add more olive oil (or lemon juice) if necessary. Set aside.

MUSHROOM AND FENNEL

2 fennel bulbs

1 lb/450 g button or cremini
mushrooms

3 sprigs fresh thyme

2 Tbsp olive oil

1 recipe Simple Vinaigrette
(see above)

½ lb/225 g mixed greens

Salt and pepper

1. Assemble, prepare, and measure ingredients. Quarter and slice fennel bulbs approximately ½ inch/1 cm thick. Chop fronds and discard stalks. Rinse, dry, and halve mushrooms. Pick thyme leaves from stalks and discard stalks. Preheat oven to 500°F/260°C.

2. In a bowl, toss fennel and mushrooms with thyme and olive oil. Season with salt and pepper. Spread out on a baking sheet and roast for 20 minutes, untouched, or until browned and tender.

3. Toss warm vegetables with Simple Vinaigrette and allow to cool completely.

4. To serve, combine cooled roasted vegetables with mixed greens and divide among four plates.

BEET AND CARROT

1 lb/450 g beets

1 lb/450 g carrots

1 tsp cumin seeds

2 Tbsp olive oil

1 recipe Simple Vinaigrette
(see above)

½ lb/225 g mixed greens

Salt and pepper

1. Assemble, prepare, and measure ingredients. Peel and slice beets approximately ½ inch/1 cm thick. Peel and slice carrots approximately ½ inch/1 cm thick. Preheat oven to 500°F/260°C.

2. In a bowl, toss beets and carrots with cumin and olive oil. Season with salt and pepper. Spread out on a baking sheet and roast for 20 minutes, untouched, or until browned and tender.

3. Toss warm vegetables with Simple Vinaigrette and allow to cool completely.

4. To serve, combine cooled roasted vegetables with mixed greens and divide among four plates.

QUINOA TABBOULEH SALAD

Tabbouleh salad is often made with cracked wheat. This version uses quinoa, a nutritional powerhouse that isn't a grain at all but a seed. While it isn't the Middle Eastern classic, this tabbouleh features the same refreshing spicy flavors as the original. Try it topped with slices of pan-fried halloumi cheese.

MAKES 4 SERVINGS

2 large tomatoes

1 shallot

1 bunch flat-leaf parsley

1 sprig fresh mint

1 lemon

¼ cup/60 mL pine nuts

1 cup/250 mL quinoa

2 tsp allspice

⅓ cup/80 mL olive oil

Salt and ground black pepper

1. Assemble, prepare, and measure ingredients. Dice tomatoes. Mince shallot. Finely chop parsley stalks and leaves, and mint leaves. Juice lemon and measure 3 tablespoons of juice.

2. Place pine nuts in a small nonstick pan and lightly toast over medium heat for about 2 minutes, until they release their nutty scent. Be careful not to burn them. Remove from heat and let cool in the pan.

3. Bring 2 cups/500 mL salted water to a boil in a small saucepan over high heat. Add quinoa, cover, turn down heat to low, and simmer for 15–20 minutes, or until quinoa forms little "tails." Remove from heat. If there is any remaining water, drain quinoa in a fine-mesh sieve. Set aside, uncovered, in saucepan or sieve.

4. Meanwhile, in a large bowl, toss together tomatoes and shallots with lemon juice. Sprinkle with allspice. Mix in parsley and mint. Stir in olive oil. Season with salt and pepper.

5. Stir quinoa into tomato-parsley mixture. Serve topped with toasted pine nuts.

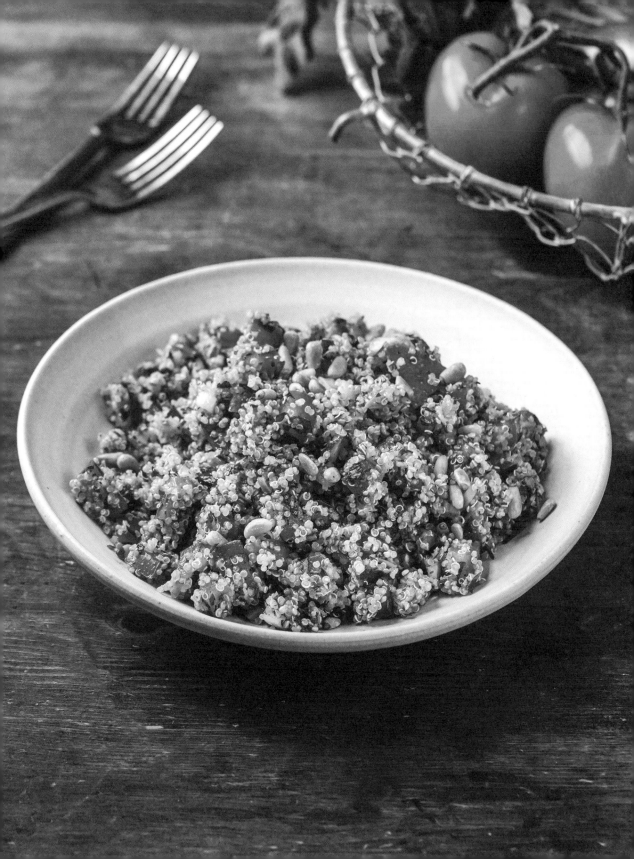

SHAVED BRUSSELS SPROUTS WITH PECORINO AND PINE NUTS

Brussels sprouts take on a whisper-light and subtle character when they are shaved. If your knife skills are in the pro league, it can be meditative to stand and chop, chop, chop. But for those of us with less-than-professional skills, the fine blade of a food processor is our best friend for this recipe.

MAKES 4 SERVINGS

1 lb/450 g Brussels sprouts

1 oz/30 g Pecorino cheese

1 lemon

½ cup/125 mL pine nuts

¼ cup/60 mL olive oil

Salt and pepper

1. Assemble, prepare, and measure ingredients. Discard any brown or yellow leaves from Brussels sprouts. Using a box grater, microplane grater, or the finest slicing blade of a food processor, shave sprouts as finely as possible. Grate Pecorino very finely. You want flakes, not chunks. Juice lemon.

2. Place pine nuts in a small nonstick pan and lightly toast over medium heat until they release their nutty scent, 1–2 minutes. Be careful not to burn them. Remove from heat and let cool in the pan.

3. In a large bowl, toss shaved Brussels sprouts with grated Pecorino, 3 tablespoons of lemon juice, and olive oil. Season with salt and pepper. Sprinkle pine nuts over top. Serve immediately.

VEGETABLES

ASIAN GREENS WITH SESAME OIL AND MISO

Miso is a paste made from fermented soybeans. It adds the savory umami note to this stir-fried side dish. This preparation will work with any dark, leafy greens, so don't worry if Asian vegetables aren't readily available. The tamari and miso are both quite salty, so don't add any salt while you're cooking.

MAKES 4 SERVINGS

1 lime

1 garlic clove

2 green onions

1 lb/450 g gai lan (Chinese broccoli) or bok choi

2 Tbsp tamari

1 Tbsp miso paste

1 tsp toasted sesame oil

1 Tbsp peanut oil

1. Assemble, prepare, and measure ingredients. Zest and juice lime. Mince garlic. Thinly slice green and white parts of green onions and place in separate piles. Trim tough bottoms from gai lan (or bok choi) and slice the rest into bite-sized pieces.

2. Combine lime zest, 1 tablespoon of lime juice, tamari, miso, and sesame oil in a small bowl. Set aside.

3. In a large wok or sauté pan over medium heat, warm peanut oil until rippling but not smoking. Stir in garlic and whites from green onions. Add gai lan (or bok choi) and cook, stirring constantly, until tender, 5 minutes. Stir in sesame-miso sauce and cook, without stirring, for another 2 minutes.

4. Transfer greens and juices from wok or pan to a serving platter, and scatter greens from green onions over top. Serve piping hot.

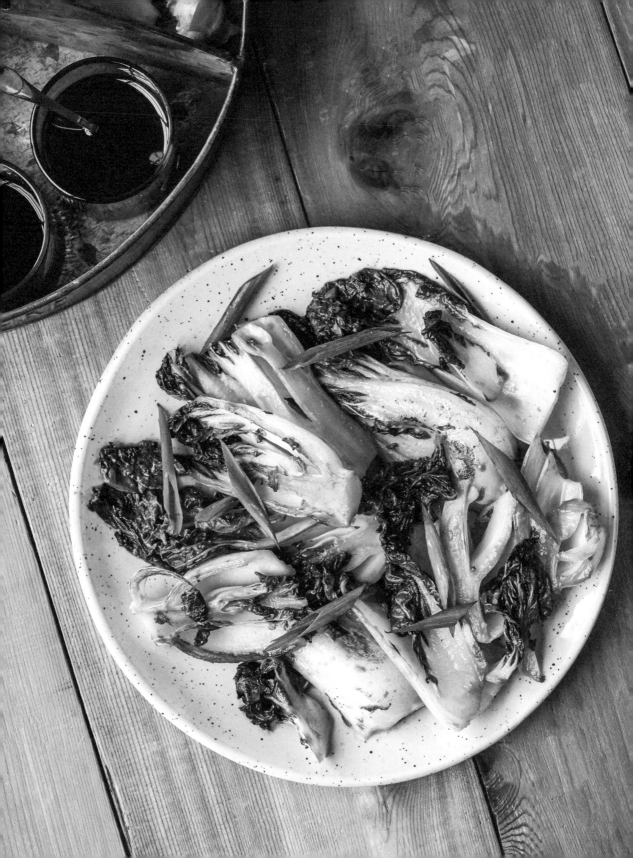

BRAISED LEEKS AND MUSHROOMS WITH PANCETTA

Leeks braised in chicken stock take on a lovely natural sweetness, offset here by earthy mushrooms and salty pancetta. Take your time so the leeks are very tender. Serve this as a light meal by itself or as an excellent side dish for unadorned fish or poultry.

MAKES 4 SERVINGS

4 oz/100 g pancetta

2 leeks, white and light green parts

1 lb/450 g mixed mushrooms

1 lemon

2 sprigs fresh thyme

1 tsp olive oil

¾ cup/175 mL chicken stock or Chicken Broth, Traditional-style (page 189)

Salt and pepper

1. Assemble, prepare, and measure ingredients. Chop pancetta. Trim tough green ends from leeks, rinse leeks very well, and cut into large pieces. Trim, rinse, and quarter mushrooms. Zest lemon. Pick thyme leaves from stalks and discard stalks.

2. In a large, heavy skillet over medium heat, warm olive oil and cook pancetta until it is beginning to crisp and fat has rendered, about 5 minutes. Add leeks and cook, stirring often, for about 7 minutes, or until softened. Transfer leeks and pancetta to a bowl and set aside.

3. Place mushrooms in fat remaining in skillet. Cook over medium heat until they release their liquid and are beginning to brown, about 5 minutes. Stir in 2 tablespoons of thyme and 1 tablespoon of lemon zest. Season generously with salt and pepper.

4. Return pancetta and leeks to skillet. Add chicken stock and bring to a boil. Turn down heat and simmer, uncovered, for 20 minutes, or until most of the liquid has been absorbed. Season with salt and pepper.

5. Divide among four individual bowls and serve hot.

BRUSSELS SPROUTS
WITH DIJON GARLIC BUTTER

You need a pile of very finely sliced Brussels sprouts for the best results in this recipe. It takes patience and good knife skills, but it's worth it. You could also use the slicing blade of a food processor, but don't use the grating or shredding blades— they shred too finely. This preparation works well with Savoy cabbage, too.

MAKES 4 SERVINGS

1 garlic clove

1 green onion

6 sprigs flat-leaf parsley

1 lb/450 g Brussels sprouts

¼ cup/60 mL butter, at room temperature

2 Tbsp Dijon or grainy mustard

Salt and pepper

1. Assemble, prepare, and measure ingredients. Mince garlic and green onion. Trim root ends of Brussels sprouts, then slice the rest into fine ribbons by hand or with a food processor. Pick parsley leaves from stalks, discard stalks, and chop leaves roughly.

2. In a small bowl, mash butter with garlic, green onions, and mustard. Season generously with salt and pepper. Cover and refrigerate for an hour before using.

3. In a large skillet set over medium-high heat, melt half the flavored butter. Drop in handfuls of Brussels sprouts, stirring as they cook down and adding more until they're all in the skillet (be careful not to crowd the pan). Sauté for 5–7 minutes, or until edges are golden brown. Stir in remaining butter, just to melt. Season with salt and pepper.

4. Transfer Brussels sprouts to a serving dish, scatter parsley over top, and serve.

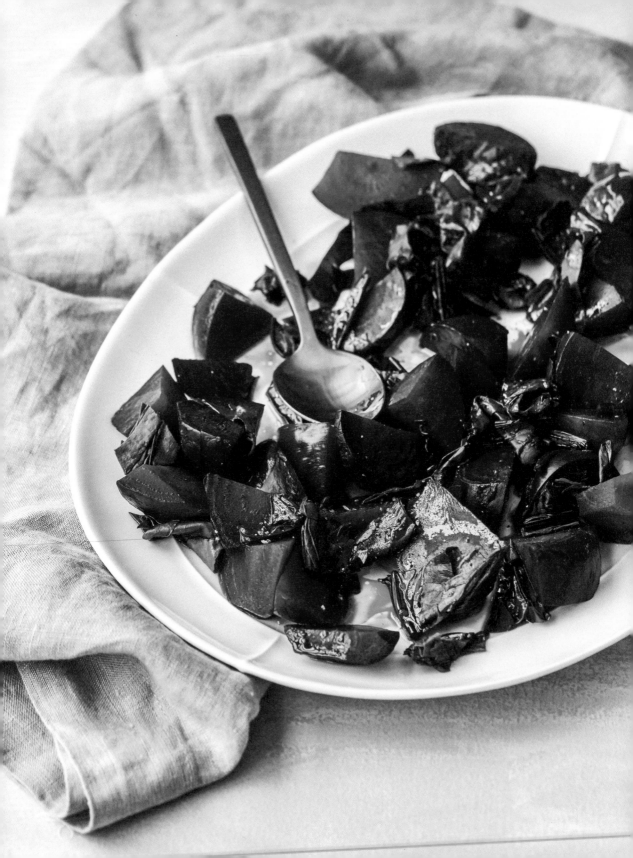

BEETS AND
THEIR GREENS

Serving beets with their greens is very pleasing, in a whole-food-is-best kind of way. The idea for this side dish came from Toronto chef Jamie Kennedy, who is a genius when it comes to perfectly subtle approaches to food. Beets are naturally sweet. The tamari gives some umami flavor to balance things out.

MAKES 4 SERVINGS

Beet greens from 1–2 bunches

8 small–medium beets

1 Tbsp apple cider vinegar

1 tsp tamari

3 Tbsp olive oil

Salt and pepper

1. Assemble, prepare, and measure ingredients. Wash beet greens. Preheat oven to 350°F/180°C.

2. Scrub beets, place in a baking dish just large enough to hold them without crowding, cover tightly with aluminum foil, and roast for 90 minutes, or until fork-tender. Allow to cool enough to handle, then peel and slice into rounds.

3. Bring a small saucepan of salted water to a boil over high heat, add beet greens, and blanch for 5 minutes. Drain well, squeezing out all the water. Chop greens.

4. In a small bowl, stir together vinegar and tamari. Arrange beet slices on a platter and dress with vinegar-tamari mixture. Scatter beet greens over top. Drizzle everything with olive oil and season with salt and pepper. Serve.

GREENS WITH COCONUT MILK

These greens are warming and filling and complement ham or roast chicken. The aromatic ginger and garlic pack a flavor wallop, softened by luscious coconut milk and brightened with lime. You can substitute gai lan (Chinese broccoli), bok choi, or tung choi for the collard greens.

MAKES 4 SERVINGS

2 shallots

2 garlic cloves

1-inch/2.5 cm piece ginger

1 bunch collard greens

2 Tbsp grapeseed oil

1 can (14 oz/400 mL) full-fat
   coconut milk

2 tsp lime juice

Salt and pepper

1. Assemble, prepare, and measure ingredients. Coarsely chop shallots. Mince garlic. Grate ginger. Chop collard greens into ribbons.

2. In a large skillet over medium heat, warm grapeseed oil. Add shallots, garlic, and ginger, and cook until aromatic, about 5 minutes. Season with salt and pepper.

3. Add coconut milk and heat until steaming. Add collard greens and cook until greens are wilted and coconut milk reduces and forms a film on them, about 12 minutes.

4. Transfer greens to a serving dish, pour in lime juice, and toss gently. Taste and adjust seasoning with more salt and pepper. Serve immediately.

GRILLED BROCCOLI
WITH CHILI-GARLIC OIL

The key to success in this recipe is cooking the components separately.
Gently infuse the garlic and chilies in olive oil—poaching them, really—
then sear the broccoli over blazing heat. The broccoli will be perfectly tender-crisp,
and you won't have bitter little pieces of charred garlic to contend with.

MAKES 4 SERVINGS

1 lb/450 g broccoli
2 garlic cloves
2 red chilies, mild or hot
1 lemon
5 Tbsp olive oil, divided
Salt and pepper

1. Assemble, prepare, and measure ingredients. Separate broccoli into florets with some stem attached. Slice garlic thinly. Slice chilies thinly. Cut lemon into wedges.

2. Fill a large bowl with ice water. Bring a large pot of salted water to a boil over high heat, add broccoli, and blanch for 3 minutes. Drain broccoli and plunge it into ice water to stop cooking. Drain again and spread out in a single layer on a clean tea towel to dry completely.

3. Warm 3 tablespoons of olive oil in a small saucepan over medium-low heat. Add garlic and chilies. Season with salt and pepper. Turn down heat to low and stir for 3–5 minutes to combine flavors. Do not allow garlic to turn dark brown. Remove from heat and set aside.

4. Toss broccoli with 2 tablespoons of olive oil. Season with salt and pepper. Heat an ungreased grill pan or heavy cast iron skillet until very hot, add a handful of broccoli, and cook, without stirring, until charred in places, about 4 minutes. Transfer cooked broccoli to a large bowl. Repeat with remaining broccoli, cooking it in batches and being careful not to crowd the pan.

5. Toss broccoli with chili-garlic oil and season with salt and pepper. Divide among four plates and serve with wedges of lemon.

ONION SOUP
WITH EMMENTHAL

The gloriously deep-brown onions in this recipe are a perfect example of
how roasting and caramelizing bring out the natural sweetness in foods without
added sugar. The slow cooking requires patience, but you can make this in
a slow-cooker or quick pressure-cooker, if you prefer. A generous quantity
of grated cheese tops this yummy, rich soup.

MAKES 4 SERVINGS

2½ lb/1 kg yellow onions

2 garlic cloves

4 oz/100 g Emmenthal or
Gruyere cheese

¼ cup/60 mL butter

1 Tbsp Dijon mustard

¾ cup/180 mL white wine or
sherry

2 quarts/2 L chicken stock or
Chicken Broth, Traditional-
style (page 189)

2 tsp sherry vinegar

Salt and pepper

1. Assemble, prepare, and measure ingredients. Slice onions
   very thinly (a food processor is a great time-saver for this).
   Mince garlic. Grate cheese.

2. In a heavy-bottomed enameled cast iron pot or other large
   heavy saucepan with a lid, melt butter over medium-high
   heat. Stir in onions and garlic. Season with salt and pepper. Cook, stirring frequently, for about 5 minutes, or until
   onions start to brown. Turn down heat to as low as possible
   and cook, uncovered, for 45–60 minutes, stirring every so
   often. If onions are drying out, add a tablespoon of water so
   they don't burn.

3. When you have a thick, dark-brown layer of onions and
   garlic, stir in mustard, followed by white wine (or sherry).
   Increase heat to medium-high and cook until liquid has
   reduced almost entirely, about 5 minutes. Add stock, bring
   to a boil, turn down heat, and simmer, partially covered, for
   about 30 minutes.

4. To serve, season with salt and pepper and add vinegar. Ladle
   soup into four deep bowls. Divide grated cheese into four
   stacks, compress them as if you're making a loose snowball,
   and place gently atop soup. Some cheese will sink and some
   will float. Best served piping hot!

PAN-ROASTED LITTLE TOMATOES WITH BASIL RIBBONS

This easy and delicious recipe looks as lovely as it tastes. Because fresh basil ribbons are added to the tomatoes while they're still warm, the basil doesn't lose its gorgeous green color or distinctive flavor. Try doubling this recipe and puree half to use as a condiment or in sauces. This is a perfect side dish for roast chicken.

MAKES 4 SERVINGS

1 lb/450 g grape or cherry tomatoes
1 garlic clove
Small handful basil leaves
1 Tbsp butter
1 Tbsp olive oil
Salt and pepper

1. Assemble, prepare, and measure ingredients. Halve tomatoes. Mince garlic. Stack basil leaves and slice into thin ribbons.

2. In a heavy-bottomed sauté pan over medium heat, melt butter with olive oil for about 2 minutes, or until a foam forms. Add tomatoes and garlic and season with salt and pepper. Stir for about 30 seconds, then turn down heat to low and cook, uncovered, for 15–20 minutes, or until tomatoes have given off most of their liquid and caramelized slightly.

3. Transfer warm tomatoes to a serving bowl, scatter basil ribbons over top, and serve immediately with a generous spoonful of pan juices.

PIPERADE

Zucchini is not always found in a classic piperade, but this version is inspired by Julia Child, whose *Mastering the Art of French Cooking* redefined many of the standards. You'll always find onions, garlic, and bell peppers in this Provencal side dish, though, along with generous amounts of olive oil for both cooking and finishing.

MAKES 4 SERVINGS

2 yellow onions

2 garlic cloves

1 lb/450 g zucchini

2 red bell peppers

1 yellow or orange bell pepper

4 sprigs fresh basil

3 Tbsp olive oil, divided

Salt and pepper

1. Assemble, prepare, and measure ingredients. Slice onions. Mince garlic. Trim stalk ends from zucchini and cut the rest into ½-inch/1 cm wide batons. Trim and seed peppers, and cut into ½-inch/1 cm slices. Stack basil leaves and slice into thin ribbons (chiffonade).

2. Warm 1 tablespoon of olive oil in a large sauté pan over medium heat. Cook onions, stirring occasionally, until translucent and golden brown, 12–15 minutes. Season with salt and pepper.

3. Add remaining 2 tablespoons of olive oil and garlic. Stir in zucchini and peppers. Season with salt and pepper. Cook for another 12–15 minutes, mostly undisturbed to allow vegetables to brown but not singe. Continue to cook if there is too much liquid; the vegetables should be juicy, not wet.

4. Transfer piperade to a serving platter and scatter basil over top. Drizzle with another spoonful of olive oil, if you like. Serve hot or at room temperature.

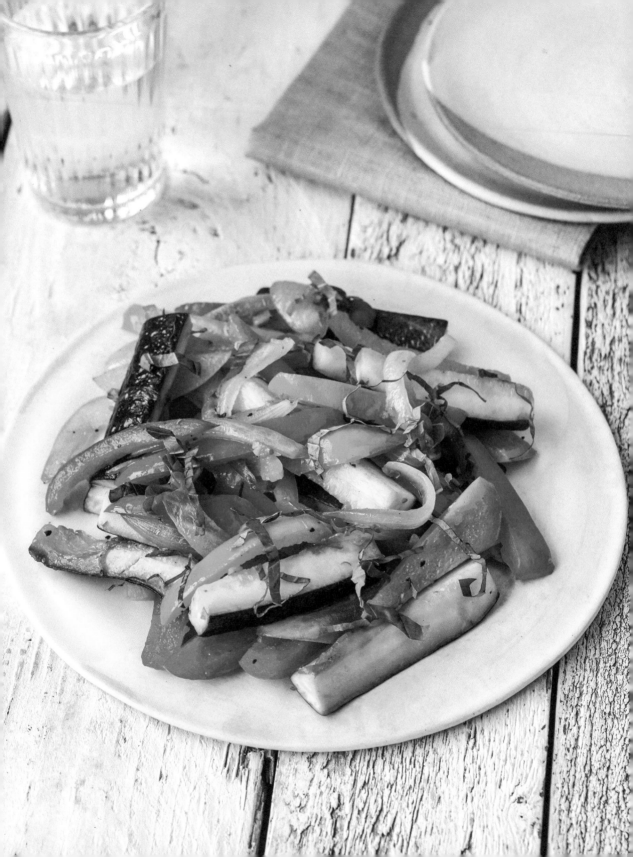

RAPINI WITH CHILI AND GARLIC

Slightly bitter, with some chewiness, rapini provides a good palette for strong Mediterranean flavors. Sometimes I add a few anchovies packed in olive oil or a few olives (not canned) with the garlic and chili for extra pungency. Rapini contains soluble fiber, which slows digestion and helps to manage insulin levels. If you can't find it, use the equivalent weight of broccolini. This can be served as a satisfying main dish or as an accompaniment.

MAKES 4 SERVINGS

1 lb/450 g rapini

2 garlic cloves

¼ cup (60 mL) olive oil

Dried chili flakes to taste

½ lemon

Salt and pepper

1. Assemble, prepare, and measure ingredients. Trim off tough stalk ends of rapini and roughly chop leaves. Mince garlic.

2. Bring a large pot of salted water to a boil over high heat, add rapini, and blanch for 2–4 minutes, or just until it changes color. Drain, spread rapini on a clean tea towel to dry thoroughly, and set aside.

3. In a large, heavy skillet over medium-high heat, warm olive oil until rippling but not smoking. Add garlic and dried chili flakes and stir for 30 seconds. Add rapini and season with salt and pepper. Pour in ¼ cup/60 mL water and cook, stirring, until rapini wilts and most of the water is gone, about 4 minutes.

4. Transfer rapini to a serving platter and squeeze juice from lemon over top. Season with more salt and pepper or chili flakes. Add another drizzle of olive oil, if you like. Serve immediately or at room temperature.

SAAG PANEER

In Hindi, saag paneer means "greens with cottage cheese." Paneer is a fresh cheese resembling cottage cheese in both appearance and flavor. Saag paneer is a popular side dish in Indian cuisine and redolent with the spices and flavors used in curries.

MAKES 4 SERVINGS

1 lb/450 g spinach

1 lb/450 g paneer

1 yellow onion

2 garlic cloves

2-inch/5 cm piece ginger

1 green chili

1 lemon

2 Tbsp ghee

1 tsp chili powder or cayenne pepper

1 tsp ground turmeric

1 tsp garam masala

Salt and pepper

1. Assemble, prepare, and measure ingredients. Rinse and chop spinach. Cube paneer. Dice onion. Roughly chop garlic, ginger, and chili. Place onions, garlic, ginger, and chili in a food processor and puree. Quarter lemon.

2. In a large nonstick skillet over medium-high heat, cook spinach very quickly in water still clinging to leaves after rinsing. Remove spinach from skillet and allow to cool. When cool enough to handle, squeeze out any residual liquid.

3. In a clean large skillet over medium-high heat, melt ghee. Add chili powder (or cayenne) and turmeric and stir for 1 minute to allow spices to bloom. Add paneer and sauté for 2 minutes, until browned on all sides. Transfer paneer to a platter, leaving spices in skillet.

4. Return skillet to medium heat. Add onion mixture and cook for 5–7 minutes, stirring occasionally, until very soft and golden brown. Stir in cooked spinach. Season with garam masala, and salt and pepper. Stir in cooked paneer to warm through.

5. Divide saag paneer among four individual bowls and serve with lemon wedges on the side.

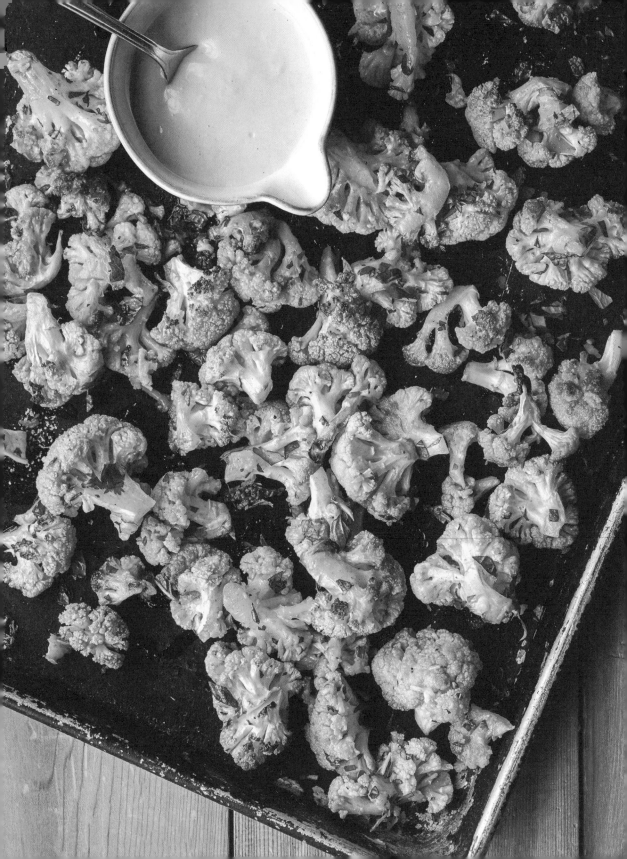

ROASTED CAULIFLOWER WITH TURMERIC AND TAHINI SAUCE

When cauliflower is roasted, it takes on a wonderful nutty character. Dipped in or drizzled with tahini sauce, this roasted cauliflower is a meal in itself but it also works well as a side dish. If you have vegetable-haters in your life, try serving them this recipe. They may find they love cauliflower!

MAKES 4–8 SERVINGS, AS A MAIN OR SIDE DISH

CAULIFLOWER

2 heads cauliflower

3 sprigs fresh cilantro

2 sprigs fresh mint

¾ cup/180 mL olive oil

1 Tbsp cumin seeds

2 tsp ground turmeric

Salt and pepper

TAHINI SAUCE

2 garlic cloves

2–3 tsp salt

½ cup/125 mL tahini

⅓ cup/80 mL lemon juice

¼ cup/60 mL olive oil

1. Assemble, prepare, and measure ingredients. Break cauliflower into florets and spread onto two ungreased baking sheets. Roughly chop cilantro and mint. Preheat oven to 425°F/220°C.

2. For the cauliflower, pour olive oil into a small bowl, stir in cumin and turmeric, and season with salt and pepper. Spoon spiced olive oil over cauliflower and toss to coat florets evenly. Roast for about 45 minutes, checking occasionally to confirm cauliflower isn't burning. Do not turn cauliflower unless you want even browning. If you ask me, it's more interesting to have a darker brown side—and it's less work for you!

3. For the tahini sauce, place garlic cloves in a mortar or on a wooden board. Add salt, 1 teaspoon at a time, and use the pestle or flat side of a knife to break down garlic and make a paste. In a small bowl, stir this garlic paste with tahini, lemon juice, ¼ cup/60 mL water, and olive oil. Set aside.

4. Toss roasted cauliflower with chopped herbs, transfer to a serving platter or individual bowls, and serve with tahini sauce on the side.

THAI VEGETABLE CURRY

While you're unlikely to find sweetcorn kernels in an authentic Thai recipe, this tasty innovation provides crunch and sweetness to contrast with the meaty chickpeas and mushrooms. Consider this recipe a Thai-inspired main dish for hungry surfers—of either the sea or the World Wide Web.

MAKES 4 SERVINGS

1 yellow onion

2 garlic cloves

½ lb/225 g white or brown mushrooms

1-inch/2.5 cm piece ginger

1 Thai red chili

1 lime

1 large bunch kale

1 bunch Thai or regular basil

1 Tbsp olive oil

1 cup/250 mL corn kernels, fresh or frozen

1 can (19 oz/540 mL) chickpeas

1 can (14 oz/400 mL) full-fat coconut milk

2 lemongrass stalks

1 Tbsp mild green curry paste

2 Tbsp tamari

1 Tbsp Thai fish sauce

Salt and black pepper

1. Assemble, prepare, and measure ingredients. Finely chop onion. Mince garlic. Halve mushrooms. Grate ginger. Thinly slice chili pepper. Juice lime. Discard kale stalks and slice leaves. Pick basil leaves from stalks and roughly chop.

2. In a large, heavy-bottomed skillet over medium heat, warm olive oil. Add onions and garlic. Cook, stirring, for about 5 minutes, or until onions start to color. Stir in mushrooms, ginger, chili, 2 tablespoons of lime juice, kale, corn, chickpeas, coconut milk, lemongrass, and curry paste. Bring mixture to a boil, then turn down heat to a simmer for 25 minutes, stirring once or twice.

3. Remove curry from heat and discard lemongrass. Stir in tamari and fish sauce, taste, and adjust seasoning with salt and pepper.

4. Transfer curry to a serving bowl or divide among four individual bowls. Serve hot, garnished with basil.

ZUCCHINI PARMIGIANA

Sometimes it doesn't matter what kind of Parmesan you use, if it's there for texture more than flavor. This is not one of those times. Here, each of the ingredients plays a co-starring role in the finished casserole, which resembles a lasagna made with zucchini. Use the best Parmigiano-Reggiano or Grana Padano you can afford.

MAKES 4–6 SERVINGS

1 can (28 oz/796 mL) whole
    tomatoes
1 yellow onion
2½ lb/1 kg zucchini
4 oz/100 g Parmigiano-
    Reggiano cheese
5 Tbsp butter
3 Tbsp olive oil
2 tsp red pepper flakes
Salt and pepper

1. Assemble, prepare, and measure ingredients. Chop tomatoes, reserving juices. Halve onion. Slice zucchini lengthwise into slices about the width of a lasagna noodle. Grate Parmesan.

2. In a skillet over medium heat, simmer tomatoes with onion, butter, and salt and pepper for 30–40 minutes, or until sauce has thickened.

3. While tomato sauce is still cooking, preheat oven to 450°F/230°C. Arrange zucchini slices in a single layer on two baking sheets. Drizzle with olive oil, sprinkle with red pepper flakes, and season with salt and pepper. Roast for 10 minutes.

4. Remove zucchini from oven. Turn down oven to 375°F/190°C. Allow zucchini slices to cool on pans until they release their liquid. Pour off their liquid.

5. Spoon a third of the tomato sauce into the bottom of a 13- × 9-inch/2 L baking dish. Cover with a third of the zucchini slices, and cover them with a third of the Parmesan. Repeat layering twice, ending with Parmesan. Bake for 30 minutes, or until bubbly and brown on top.

6. Remove from oven and allow to cool for 20 minutes before slicing. Serve warm.

POULTRY: CHICKEN, DUCK, AND TURKEY

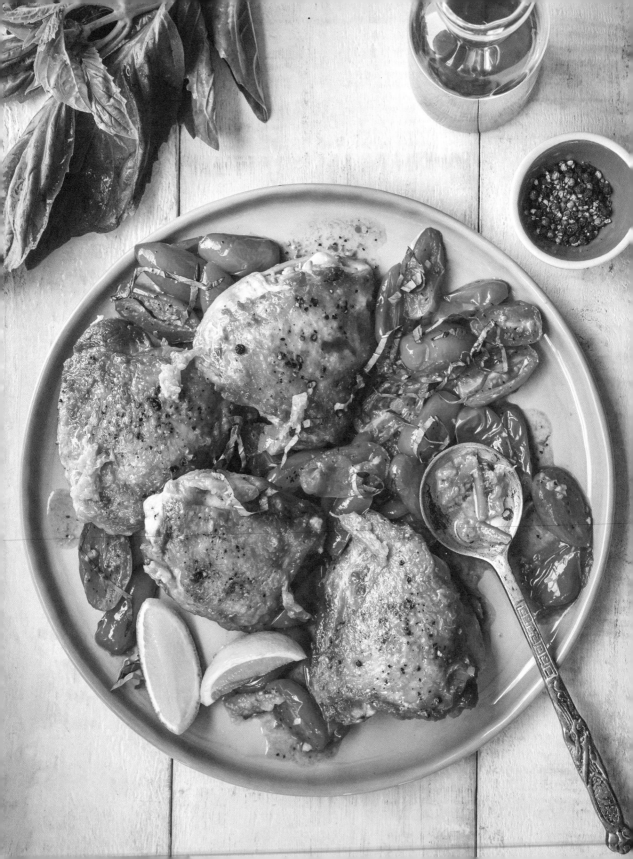

CHICKEN THIGHS
WITH PRESERVED LEMON

This is a magical recipe where the chicken fat works wonders—if you are patient. Preserved lemon balances the fat perfectly, and the spritz of fresh lemon juice at the end will wake up your taste buds. This dish is particularly good with a dark green leafy vegetable, such as kale or collard greens, or with Pan-roasted Little Tomatoes with Basil Ribbons (page 97).

MAKES 4 SERVINGS

8 bone-in, skin-on chicken thighs
1 preserved lemon
1 lemon
1 Tbsp olive oil
Salt and pepper

1. Assemble, prepare, and measure ingredients. Season chicken skin liberally with salt and pepper. Slice preserved lemon rind into fine slivers. Quarter fresh lemon.

2. In a large, heavy skillet, preferably cast iron, warm olive oil over medium heat until it shimmers. Add chicken thighs, skin side down, and allow to cook undisturbed for 30 minutes. Turn down heat if chicken skin starts to burn, but otherwise leave fat to render and skin to crisp up.

3. When skin is crisp and golden, turn chicken over. Stir in preserved lemon rind, mixing it well into the delicious pan juices. Cook for another 12–15 minutes, or until juices run clear when you pierce chicken with the tip of a knife.

4. Transfer chicken to a serving platter, drizzle with pan juices, and serve with lemon wedges on the side.

CHICKEN BREASTS POACHED IN ROSÉ

This delicious recipe is easy, with only a few key ingredients. It's also a perfect make-ahead dish—and leftovers work beautifully sliced over salad. And the rosé sauce doubles as a salad dressing: just thin it with a little lemon juice or tone down the mustard with some olive oil. Cook's choice!

MAKES 4 SERVINGS

6 garlic cloves

6 basil leaves

¼ cup/60 mL olive oil

1 cup/250 mL rosé or
    zinfandel wine

2 lb/900 g boneless chicken
    breasts

1 Tbsp Dijon or grainy
    mustard

Salt and pepper

1. Assemble, prepare, and measure ingredients. Smash garlic. Roughly tear basil leaves.

2. In a heavy-bottomed saucepan just large enough to hold the chicken breasts snugly, warm olive oil over medium heat. Add garlic and stir with olive oil for 1 minute, or until aromatic. Be careful not to let garlic brown. Stir in wine and season with salt and pepper.

3. Add chicken and enough water, if necessary, so chicken breasts are completely covered in liquid. Bring to a boil, turn down heat to low, cover, and simmer for 15–18 minutes, or until internal temperature of chicken is 160°F/71°C. Remove from heat and allow chicken to cool in its poaching liquid.

4. Once cool, place chicken on a cutting surface. Strain 2 cups/500 mL poaching liquid into a glass measuring cup. In a small saucepan over medium-high heat, reduce strained liquid to about 1 cup/250 mL. Stir in mustard. Taste and adjust seasoning with salt and pepper.

5. Thinly slice chicken and arrange on a serving platter or individual plates. To serve, drizzle with wine-mustard sauce and scatter basil over top.

CHICKEN LIVERS WITH SHERRY AND CREAM

This is an elegant preparation, with a Spanish-influenced addition of sherry. A fine, dark oloroso is the perfect fortified wine to sip on while you cook this— but ordinary cooking sherry is just fine for the actual recipe!

MAKES 4 SERVINGS

1 lb/450 g chicken livers

1 yellow onion

2 garlic cloves

2 sprigs fresh flat-leaf or curly parsley

1 sprig fresh thyme

2 Tbsp olive oil

¼ cup/60 mL chicken stock or Chicken Broth, Traditional-style (page 189)

2 Tbsp dry sherry

2 Tbsp crème fraîche or heavy cream

Salt and pepper

1. Assemble, prepare, and measure ingredients. Clean chicken livers, trimming off any sinew. Finely chop onion. Mince garlic. Pick leaves from parsley and thyme sprigs and roughly chop leaves.

2. In a heavy skillet over medium-high heat, warm olive oil until it shimmers. Add chicken livers and sear on all sides, about 5 minutes. Transfer livers to a plate. Place onions and garlic in skillet and cook for 6–8 minutes, until softened but not browned.

3. Add stock and sherry, scraping up any brown bits in the skillet with a wooden spoon. Bring to a boil and then turn down heat to a simmer. Return chicken livers to skillet and simmer, uncovered, for 5 minutes. They should still be pale pink in the center. Remove from heat.

4. Arrange chicken livers on a serving platter. Stir crème fraîche (or cream) into pan juices and pour over the chicken. Season with salt and pepper. Scatter parsley and thyme over top before serving.

MEDITERRANEAN ONE-PAN CHICKEN AND VEGETABLES

Who doesn't love a one-pan dinner? This iteration combines bold flavors in big moves—forget teaspoons of this or pinches of that; instead use the whole bunch, the whole head, olives, AND bacon. Don't be shy about increasing the quantity of veggies: just use two baking sheets instead of one roasting pan.

MAKES 4 SERVINGS

2 small zucchinis

1 yellow onion

1 head garlic

½ lb/225 g Kalamata olives

1 bunch fresh basil

4 Tbsp olive oil, divided

½ lb/225 g bacon or sliced pancetta

8 skin-on, bone-in chicken thighs and legs (4 of each)

1 lb/450 g grape tomatoes

1 bird's eye chili

Salt and pepper

1. Assemble, prepare, and measure ingredients. Slice zucchini thickly into rounds about ½ inch/1 cm thick. Cut onion into eight wedges. Separate garlic cloves from their bulb but don't peel them. Smash garlic in its peel, then discard the peel. Remove pits from olives. Roughly chop basil leaves. Preheat oven to 350°F/180°C.

2. Line a plate with paper towels. Add 2 tablespoons olive oil to a roasting pan large enough to fit all the ingredients in one layer. Place bacon (or pancetta) in roasting pan and cook over medium-low heat for 10 minutes. Use a slotted spoon to transfer bacon (or pancetta) to plate to drain.

3. Place zucchini, onions, garlic, olives, basil, chicken, tomatoes, and chili in pan. Drizzle with the remaining 2 tablespoons of olive oil and season with salt and pepper. Toss everything together to coat well. Shake pan to settle ingredients into a (mostly) single layer. Roast, undisturbed, for 30 minutes.

4. Place bacon (or pancetta) over top of other ingredients and cook for another 15–20 minutes, or until juices run clear when chicken is pierced close to the bone.

5. Serve chicken with vegetables and bacon (or pancetta), spooning over some pan juices, if you like.

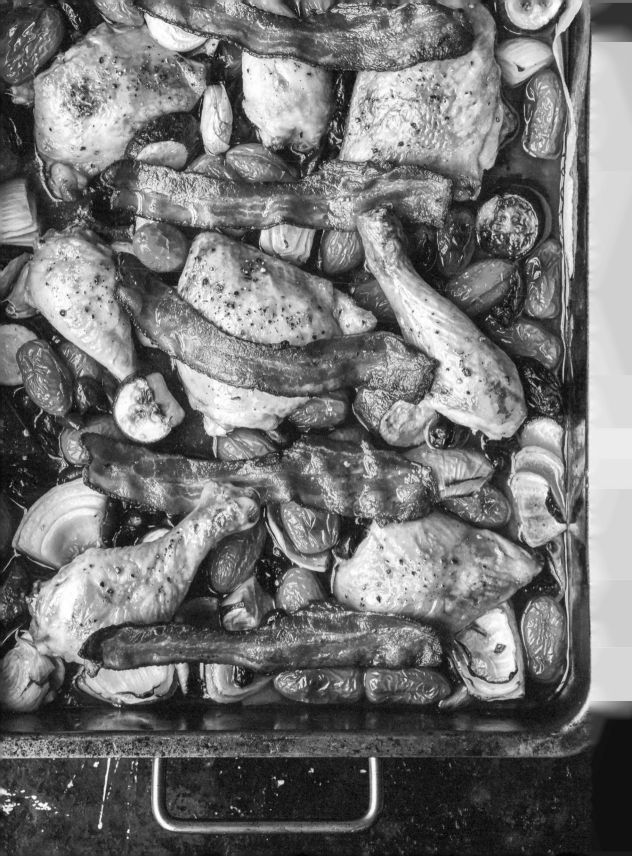

CHICKEN WITH SESAME SEED CRUST

If you love fried chicken, here is a version made extra tasty with the Asian flavors of citrus, ginger, and soy and a crunchy and salty sesame seed coating. An added bonus is the fiber from the seeds, but who's counting? This chicken is delicious with Asian Greens with Sesame Oil and Miso (page 88).

MAKES 4 SERVINGS

1½ lb/680 g boneless, skinless chicken breasts

1-inch/2.5 cm piece ginger

1 lime

6 sprigs fresh cilantro or flat-leaf parsley

½ cup/125 mL sesame seeds (white or black)

1 Tbsp grapeseed oil

1 tsp toasted sesame oil

¼ cup/60 mL butter

1 Tbsp tamari

Salt and pepper

1. Assemble, prepare, and measure ingredients. Pound chicken breasts to an even thickness of about 1 inch (2.5 cm). Grate ginger. Zest and juice lime. Roughly tear or chop cilantro (or parsley) leaves.

2. Pour sesame seeds into a shallow bowl. Season chicken with salt and pepper, then press both sides of chicken into sesame seeds. Set aside on wax or parchment paper.

3. In a large heavy skillet over medium heat, warm grapeseed and sesame oils. Cook chicken breasts for 6 minutes, then turn over and cook for another 4 minutes. (If your skillet is not large enough to hold all the chicken at once, cook it in batches.) Turn down heat if necessary to avoid burning sesame seeds. Transfer cooked chicken to a serving platter and keep warm while you make the sauce.

4. In the same skillet, melt butter. Add ginger and sauté lightly for about 30 seconds. Stir in 1 tablespoon of lime juice and the tamari and cook for 1 minute to allow flavors to blend.

5. To serve, pour sauce over chicken and sprinkle with lime zest and cilantro (or parsley). Serve immediately.

MOROCCAN CHICKEN WITH TURMERIC AND APRICOTS

This recipe contains traditional Moroccan ingredients like aromatic cream, turmeric, and dried fruit, but I've reduced the amount of fruit found in authentic North African dishes to limit the fructose content. It's not a traditional preparation, so the recipe title is a bit of a misnomer. But it certainly is delicious!

MAKES 4 SERVINGS

8 bone-in, skin-on chicken thighs
1 yellow onion
2 garlic cloves
1-inch/2.5 cm piece ginger
4½ oz/125 g dried apricots
3 Tbsp currants
3 Tbsp olive oil
½ tsp ground turmeric
½ cup/125 mL sour cream
½ cup water or chicken stock (or Chicken Broth, Traditional-style, page 189)
Salt and pepper

1. Assemble, prepare, and measure ingredients. Pat chicken thighs dry with paper towel. Dice onion. Mince garlic. Grate ginger. Cut apricots into slivers. Wash currants in warm water and drain well.

2. In a large, heavy-bottomed skillet with a lid over medium-high heat, warm olive oil until hot but not smoking. Brown chicken thighs on both sides, 5–7 minutes per side. (If your skillet is not large enough to hold all the chicken at once, cook it in batches.) Transfer cooked chicken to a platter and set aside.

3. Pour off all but 1 tablespoon of oil. Add turmeric to hot oil and stir for about 1 minute to allow it to bloom. Stir in onion and cook for about 5 minutes, or until translucent. Add garlic and ginger and cook for 2 minutes, or until aromatic. Whisk in sour cream and then water (or stock). Bring to a boil and then turn down heat to low to simmer. Add apricots and currants and season with salt and pepper.

4. Return chicken to skillet and simmer over low heat, uncovered, for 30–40 minutes, or until juices run clear when thigh is pierced close to the bone.

5. Serve in bowls and eat with spoons to catch all of the delicious sauce.

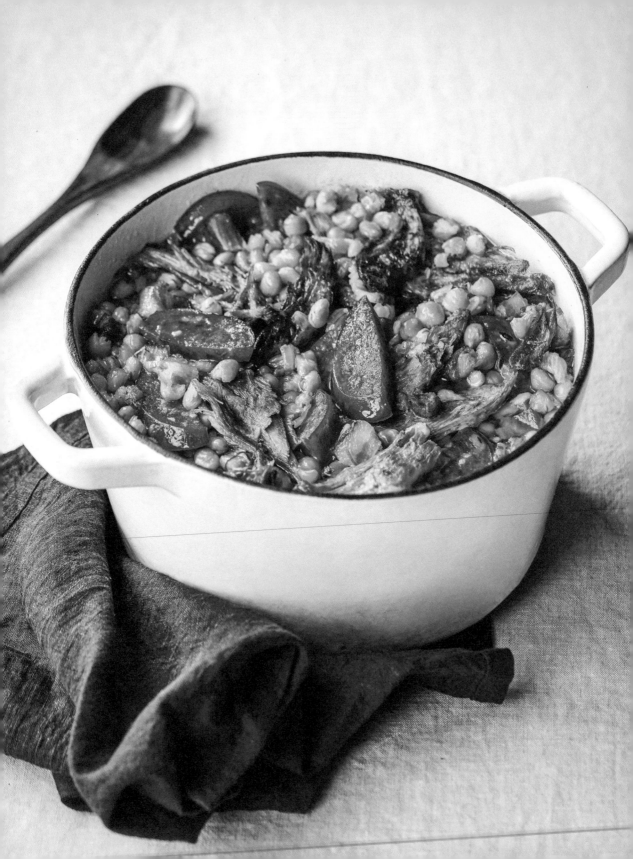

QUICK DUCK CASSOULET

Even at a couple of hours for prep and cooking time, this still qualifies as
"quick" when it comes to making cassoulet. An authentic cassoulet involves soaking
and stewing raw beans, preparing duck confit, and simmering for hours.
A few shortcuts result in something less classic but just as mouthwatering.

MAKES 4 SERVINGS

4 oz/100 g pancetta

1 yellow onion

1 can (28 oz/796 mL) navy
    beans

6 garlic cloves

4 pieces prepared duck confit

1 lb/450 g French garlic
    sausage

4 slices bacon

4 sprigs fresh flat-leaf parsley
    (optional)

5 Tbsp olive oil, divided

4 sprigs fresh thyme

1 quart/1 L chicken stock or
    Chicken Broth, Traditional-
    style (page 189)

1. Assemble, prepare, and measure ingredients. Cut pancetta
   into small cubes. Finely chop onion. Drain and rinse beans.
   Peel and smash garlic. Tear duck confit into bite-sized
   pieces. Cut sausage into ½-inch/1 cm slices. Chop bacon
   into lardons. Mince parsley (if using). Preheat oven to
   350°F/180°C.

2. Heat 3 tablespoons of olive oil in a large saucepan over
   medium heat. Add pancetta and cook for 5–7 minutes, until
   fat renders. Stir in onion and cook until softened, about
   5 minutes. Add beans, garlic, thyme sprigs, and finally
   chicken broth. Bring to a boil, turn down heat to low, and
   simmer, uncovered, for 15 minutes.

3. Butter a 13- × 9-inch/2 L baking dish. Place beans, duck
   confit, sausage, bacon, and any residual liquid from pot in
   it. Bake, uncovered, for 45 minutes, or until meat is cooked.
   Remove from oven and allow to rest for 15 minutes.

4. To serve, spoon into four individual bowls and garnish with
   parsley (if using).

TEA-BRAISED
DUCK WITH FENNEL

The grassy notes of the green tea and fennel contrast with the rich,
meaty depth of the duck. It's important to render the fat from the duck before
braising it to yield a clear and savory sauce.

MAKES 4 SERVINGS

4 large duck legs

1 small yellow onion

½ fennel bulb

1-inch/2.5 cm piece ginger

4 green tea bags or 4 tsp
   Pique Ginger Green tea
   crystals

⅓ cup + 1 tsp/85 mL white
   wine vinegar

2 tsp Chinese five-spice
   powder

Salt and pepper

1. Assemble, prepare, and measure ingredients. Season duck liberally with salt and pepper. Thinly slice onion and fennel. Grate ginger. Boil 2 cups/500 mL of water, and steep tea for 10 minutes. Preheat oven to 300°F/150°C.

2. Place duck legs in a cold roasting pan set over medium heat. Cook until fat begins to render and sizzle, about 5 minutes. Turn legs over and brown for 5 minutes. Transfer duck to a plate and set aside. Pour off all but 1 tablespoon of the fat.

3. Return pan to heat and add the ⅓ cup/80 mL vinegar, scraping up any brown bits in the pan with a wooden spoon. Simmer vinegar until reduced by half, about 5 minutes. Add onion, fennel, and ginger and cook until translucent, 5–7 minutes. Season with Chinese five-spice, and salt and pepper.

4. Return duck to pan and add enough green tea to come almost halfway up the duck. Place pan in oven and braise, uncovered, for 1 hour and 15 minutes, or until very tender.

5. Transfer duck legs to a plate and cover loosely with aluminum foil. Skim any excess fat from braising liquid. Set roasting pan on stovetop over medium-low heat and simmer braising liquid until it reduces by half and thickens, about 8 minutes. Finish sauce with 1 teaspoon vinegar.

6. To serve, unwrap duck legs and drizzle sauce over top.

TURKEY CURRY

Turkey and curry are not an obvious flavor pairing, but they are a match made in heaven! This very easy turkey curry uses cooked meat with cauliflower and tomatoes to make a complete one-pot meal. Feel free to amp up the spice by adding more curry paste if you prefer.

MAKES 4 SERVINGS

1 yellow onion

1 garlic clove

1 red bell pepper

½ head cauliflower

1 lb/450 g cooked turkey

1 Tbsp coconut oil

2–3 Tbsp curry paste (your favorite!)

1 can (15 oz/426 mL) chopped tomatoes

Salt and pepper

1. Assemble, prepare, and measure ingredients. Dice onion. Chop garlic. Seed and chop bell pepper. Break cauliflower into small florets. Cube turkey into bite-sized pieces.

2. In a medium saucepan with a lid, heat coconut oil over medium-high heat. Add onion, garlic, bell pepper, and cauliflower and sauté for 5 minutes or so, just to soften everything and brown slightly. Stir in turkey and curry paste and allow flavors to combine for 1 minute.

3. Add tomatoes with their juice and some water, if necessary, to just cover the turkey and veggies. Bring to a lively simmer and cook, partially covered, for 8–10 minutes, or until cauliflower is tender-crisp.

4. Serve in bowls.

TURKEY CHILI

If turkey chili sounds like a throwback to the days when lean meats like turkey were substituted for fattier pork and beef, fear not. This chili is actually *tastier* made with ground turkey than other ground meats, meaning that flavor is not sacrificed for health. Sweet potatoes are on the starchier side but they come with plenty of vitamins and fiber.

MAKES 4 SERVINGS

2 sweet potatoes (optional)
1 yellow onion
2 garlic cloves
1 can (14 oz/398 mL) red or
   white kidney beans
1 bunch fresh cilantro
2–4 Tbsp olive oil
1 tsp ground cumin
1 tsp smoked paprika
1 tsp chili powder
1 lb/450 g ground turkey
1 can (28 oz/796 mL) whole
   tomatoes
½ cup/125 mL full-fat sour
   cream
Lime wedges, for serving
Salt and pepper

1. Assemble, prepare, and measure ingredients. Peel and cube sweet potatoes (if using). Chop onion. Mince garlic. Rinse and drain beans. Chop cilantro stalks and leaves. If using sweet potatoes, preheat oven to 425°F/220°C and line a baking sheet with parchment paper.

2. In a mixing bowl, toss sweet potatoes with 2 tablespoons of olive oil and salt and pepper. Spread in a single layer on baking sheet and roast for 20–25 minutes, or until fork-tender. Remove from oven and set aside.

3. In a heavy-bottomed chili pot over medium heat, warm the remaining 2 tablespoons of olive oil and add onions, garlic, cumin, paprika, chili powder, and salt and pepper. Cook, stirring frequently, until onions are soft but not beginning to brown, 8–10 minutes.

4. Add ground turkey, breaking it up with a wooden spoon so you don't end up with little turkey meatballs, and cook for 15–20 minutes, or until turkey is mostly brown. Add beans and tomatoes (with their juices) and simmer for 15 minutes, breaking up tomatoes with a wooden spoon. Add roasted sweet potatoes (if using) and simmer for another 5 minutes. Taste and adjust seasoning with salt and pepper.

5. To serve, ladle chili into four individual bowls, garnish with a dollop of sour cream, and sprinkle with chopped cilantro. Offer lime wedges on the side.

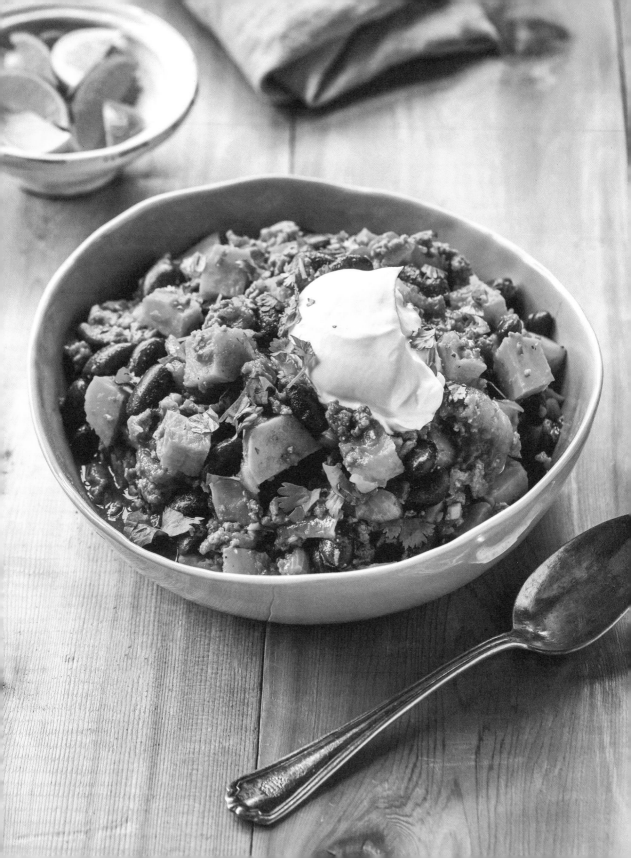

FISH AND SHELLFISH

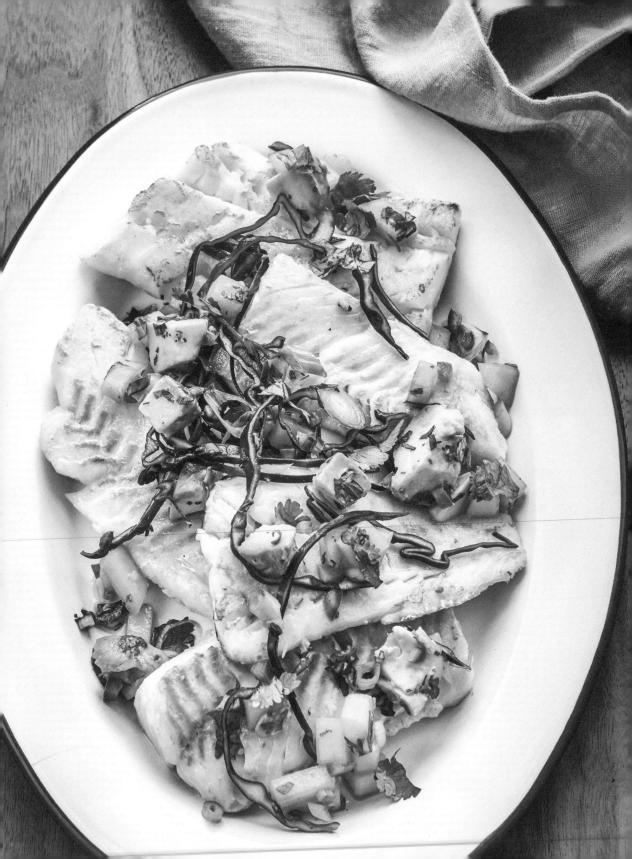

COD WITH
MANGO AVOCADO SLAW

Food that looks this beautiful awakens the appetite. The slaw is a perfect
accompaniment to meaty but mild cod, as it offers irresistible crunch, with sweet mango
and creamy avocado, all in a spicy citrus dressing to arouse your taste buds.
These ingredients are best when freshly combined so they retain their individual flavors
and textures. For a real indulgence, try this recipe with halibut.

MAKES 4 SERVINGS

1 large mango

2 avocados

½ small red cabbage

6 sprigs fresh cilantro

1 green onion

1 jalapeño pepper

1 lime

5 Tbsp olive oil, divided

1 Tbsp butter

4 (total weight of 2 lb/900 g)
   cod fillets

Ground cumin

Salt and pepper

1. Assemble, prepare, and measure ingredients. Peel and dice mango and avocados. Using a box grater or knife—a food processor shreds too coarsely for this dish—shred cabbage finely. Chop cilantro stalks and leaves. Finely chop green and white parts of green onion. Seed and mince jalapeño. Zest and juice lime. Preheat oven to 425°F/220°C.

2. In a large ovenproof skillet over medium-high heat, warm 3 tablespoons of olive oil with the butter. Season cod with salt and pepper and place in skillet, leaving space between fillets. Sear for 3 minutes, then turn fillets over and transfer skillet to oven for 5 minutes to finish cooking.

3. While cod is cooking, combine mango, avocado, cabbage, cilantro, green onion, jalapeño, lime zest and juice, pinch of cumin, and 2 tablespoons of olive oil. Season with salt and pepper.

4. Serve cod warm on individual plates with slaw on the side.

COD WITH SUNDRIED TOMATO AND PECAN CRUST

A pungent, aromatic crust makes the most of meaty, substantial cod. You'll enjoy this substitute for fried fish—no batter!—so much you may never eat old-school fish and chips again. This recipe calls for pecans, which are naturally sweet and rich, but you could substitute crushed cashews or walnuts, if you like.

MAKES 4 SERVINGS

2 oz/55 g Parmesan cheese

2 garlic cloves

10 sprigs fresh basil

1 lemon

4 (total weight 2 lb/900 g) cod fillets, skin-on

2 Tbsp olive oil, divided

10 anchovies in oil

½ cup/125 mL sundried tomatoes in oil

3½ oz/95 g crushed pecans

1 red chili pepper

Salt and pepper

1. Assemble, prepare, and measure ingredients. Roughly chop Parmesan into chunks. Roughly chop garlic. Pick basil leaves from stalks and discard stalks. Zest and juice lemon. Preheat oven to 500°F/260°C.

2. In a baking dish large enough to hold the fillets in a single layer without crowding, place cod skin-side down, drizzle with 1 tablespoon olive oil, and season with salt and pepper. Roast until fish starts to flake, 5–7 minutes, depending on thickness of fillets.

3. Meanwhile, place Parmesan, garlic, basil, lemon zest, anchovies, sundried tomatoes, pecans, and chili in a food processor. Pulse a few times to mix ingredients evenly. Add 1 tablespoon of lemon juice and 1 tablespoon of olive oil. Season with salt and pepper. Whir to a paste in the food processor.

4. Remove cod from oven. Pack a thick, even layer of coating mixture on each fillet. You may need to press slightly to get the mixture to stay together. Don't worry if some crumbs fall off. Return cod to oven and roast for another 5–7 minutes, or until coating is crisp and dark brown in places.

5. To serve, place cod on individual plates.

BAKED SALMON
WITH CAJUN SPICE

Salmon is a wonderful food choice for its higher (healthy) fat content, gorgeous color, and adaptability. Just don't overcook it, please! There is a natural sweetness to salmon that marries deliciously with a Cajun-style spicy blend. Serve this dish with a heap of sautéed greens and some quinoa.

MAKES 4 SERVINGS

2 Tbsp butter

2 Tbsp smoked paprika

1 Tbsp cayenne pepper

1 Tbsp onion powder

1 tsp dried thyme leaves

1 tsp dried oregano

1 tsp dried basil

4 (total weight 24 oz/700 g) salmon fillets

Salt and pepper

1. Assemble, prepare, and measure ingredients. Melt and cool butter. Preheat oven to 450°F/230°C. Lightly brush a baking dish large enough to hold salmon fillets in a single layer with some melted butter.

2. In a small bowl, combine paprika, cayenne, onion powder, thyme, oregano, and basil.

3. Place salmon fillets in baking dish, brush with remaining melted butter, and season with salt and pepper. Sprinkle seasoning mix evenly over fillets. Bake for 10–12 minutes, or until topping is light brown and salmon is still deep pink in center.

4. To serve, place salmon on individual plates.

MILK-POACHED SALMON WITH GREMOLATA

Milk poaching is an unusual preparation, but one that you may want to try with other types of fish or even chicken breasts. Milk is sometimes used to braise pork shoulder too. The lactose in the milk helps to tenderize the fish or meat, resulting in a velvety-soft texture and a mild, slightly nutty flavor.

MAKES 4 SERVINGS

4 (total weight 2 lb/900 g)
   fresh salmon fillets
1 garlic clove
1 lemon
½ bunch flat-leaf parsley
2–3 cups/500–750 mL 2%
   milk
1 bay leaf
1 Tbsp olive oil
Salt and pepper

1. Assemble, prepare, and measure ingredients. Using a sharp knife, cut each fillet into four and season with salt and pepper. Grate garlic. Zest lemon. Finely chop parsley.

2. Pour milk into a large skillet to a depth of about 1 inch/2.5 cm. (You may need more milk than is listed here.) Add bay leaf and heat on medium until milk is steaming but not quite boiling (no more than a simmer). Place salmon in skillet. The milk should come at least halfway up the fillets. (Warm up more milk and add to pan, if necessary.) Lower heat slightly to simmer gently for 15 minutes.

3. While salmon is cooking, stir together garlic, lemon zest, parsley, and olive oil in a small bowl for your gremolata. Set aside.

4. To serve, place fillets on individual plates and spoon gremolata over top.

POACHED SALMON
WITH LIME-DILL MAYONNAISE

Here's another approach to poaching salmon, this time in a white wine infusion. Adding fresh herbs and mustard to mayonnaise is a good kitchen trick: it tastes like you went to a lot of trouble when really you didn't! Dill and salmon are a classic pairing, but feel free to substitute any fresh herb. Basil is particularly good.

MAKES 4 SERVINGS

1 lime

1 small bunch chives

2 sprigs fresh dill

1 shallot

½ cup/125 mL white wine

1 bay leaf

4 (total weight 24 oz/700 g)
    salmon fillets

½ cup/125 mL mayonnaise

1 Tbsp Dijon mustard

Salt and pepper

1. Assemble, prepare, and measure ingredients. Zest and juice lime. Mince chives. Mince dill. Mince shallot.

2. In a wide, high-sided skillet, combine 3 cups/750 mL water and white wine, add shallots, bay leaf, and 1 teaspoon of salt, and bring to a boil over high heat. Let liquid reduce slightly for 5 minutes and remove from heat.

3. Carefully lower salmon fillets into poaching liquid, cover pan with lid, and allow salmon to poach in liquid as it cools. Check salmon after 15 minutes. It should be deep pink in the center. If it is not quite cooked, leave it to poach for 5 more minutes.

4. Transfer cooked salmon to a platter to rest for 5 minutes. Pat dry with paper towel. (If you are not serving fish right away, cover platter and refrigerate for up to 3 days.)

5. While salmon is resting, in a small bowl, combine mayonnaise with 1 teaspoon of lime zest, 1 tablespoon of lime juice, chives, dill, and mustard. Season with salt and pepper.

6. Serve salmon at room temperature. Place a fillet on each of four individual plates and top with a generous dollop of lime-dill mayonnaise.

SCALLOPS WITH PROSCIUTTO

This recipe is a good choice for special dinners or when you're entertaining. Garlicky, salty, and a little bit spicy, it's not difficult or time-consuming to prepare but it is guaranteed to get rave reviews. Rapini with Chili and Garlic (page 100) makes a perfect side dish for this recipe.

MAKES 4 SERVINGS

2 lb/900 g grape tomatoes

1 garlic clove

2 dried red chilies

6 anchovies

1 can (19 oz/540 mL) cannellini beans

1 lemon

4 Tbsp olive oil, divided

8 slices prosciutto

16 sea scallops

Salt and pepper

1. Assemble, prepare, and measure ingredients. Halve tomatoes. Mince garlic. Crumble dried chilies. Mash anchovies with a fork. Rinse and drain beans. Juice lemon. Preheat oven to 475°F/245°C.

2. Scatter tomatoes on a baking sheet, drizzle with 1 tablespoon of olive oil, season with salt and pepper, and roast for 10 minutes. Push tomatoes to one side of the baking sheet and arrange prosciutto slices in a single layer on the other. Roast for a further 10 minutes to crisp prosciutto. Remove from oven and set aside.

3. In a skillet over medium-high heat, heat 1 tablespoon of olive oil. Add garlic, chilies, and mashed anchovies. Sauté for 1 minute, then add beans and ½ cup/125 mL water. Mash beans coarsely as they warm through. Remove from heat, add a drizzle of olive oil, and season with salt and pepper. Set aside.

4. In another skillet, heat 1 tablespoon of olive oil. Season scallops with salt and pepper, add to skillet, and sear for 2 minutes, undisturbed, until burnished golden brown. Turn scallops over and cook for another 2 minutes.

5. To serve, arrange tomatoes, two slices of prosciutto, and beans on each of four individual plates. Top each one with four scallops. Sprinkle with lemon juice and a little more olive oil and season with salt and pepper.

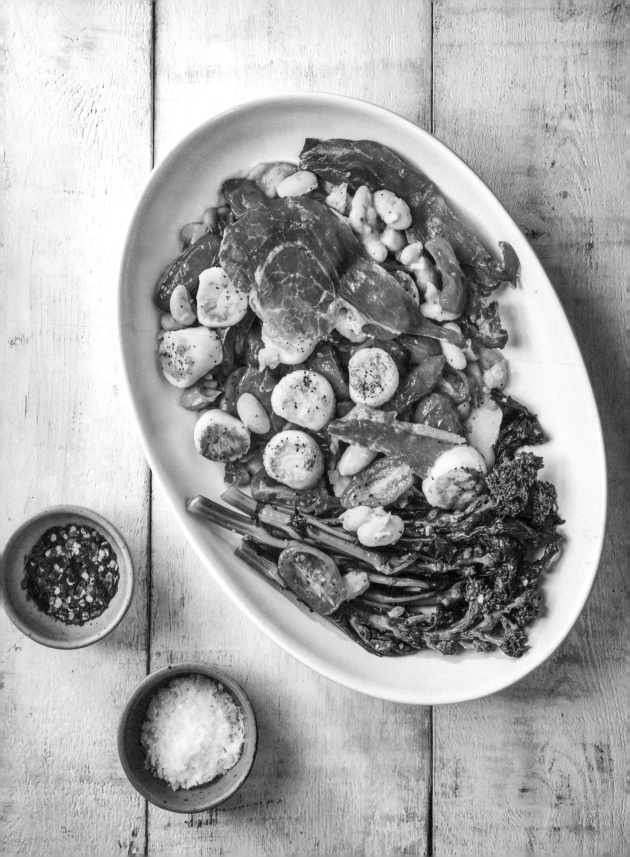

SALMON CAKES
WITH BEURRE BLANC

The revelation in this recipe is the beurre blanc, which elevates humble
fish cakes to something heavenly. Beurre blanc resembles hollandaise sauce,
but without the eggs it doesn't thicken as much. Learn to make this
elegant, adaptable sauce and you will never have a boring dinner again.

MAKES 4 SERVINGS

SALMON CAKES

1 red bell pepper

2 green onions

½ bunch flat-leaf parsley

2 eggs

2 cans (each 7½ oz/212 g)
    pink or red salmon

1 cup/250 mL almond flour

2 tsp Dijon mustard

1 Tbsp melted butter

Grapeseed oil, for frying

Salt and pepper

BEURRE BLANC

1 shallot

½ cup/125 mL butter

2 Tbsp dry white wine

2 Tbsp white wine vinegar

2 Tbsp 18% cream

Finely ground white pepper

Salt

1. Assemble, prepare, and measure ingredients. Halve bell
pepper lengthwise and discard stem and seeds. Coarsely
chop green onions. Coarsely chop parsley. Whisk eggs in a
small mixing bowl until combined. Drain cans of salmon.
Finely chop shallot, measure out 1 tablespoon, and set aside
remainder. Cube ½ cup/125 mL butter. Preheat oven to
400°F/200°C.

2. Place bell pepper skin-side up on a baking sheet and roast
for 30 minutes, or until skin begins to shrivel and blacken
slightly. Remove from oven, allow to cool slightly, and then
dice half of it. Reserve the other half for another use.

3. Combine diced bell pepper, green onions, parsley, eggs,
almond flour, mustard, and 1 tablespoon melted butter in
a mixing bowl. Use a fork to gently but thoroughly incorporate the salmon. Form mixture into four patties, set on
a plate, and refrigerate, uncovered, while you make the
beurre blanc.

4. For the beurre blanc, combine shallot, wine, and vinegar
in a small saucepan and bring to a boil over medium-high
heat. Turn down heat to medium and cook until barely any
liquid remains, 5–7 minutes. Stir in cream and pinch of
white pepper and cook for 1 minute. Add butter, 1–2 cubes

at a time, whisking continuously and waiting until butter is nearly melted before adding more. Once all butter is added and mixture is completely liquefied, remove saucepan from heat. Season sauce with salt, then strain through a fine-mesh sieve into a small bowl. Discard residual solids.

5. For the salmon cakes, heat grapeseed oil in a large, heavy skillet over medium-high heat. Cook for 4 minutes, then turn over and cook for a further 3 minutes.

6. To serve, place a salmon cake on each of four individual plates and drizzle with beurre blanc.

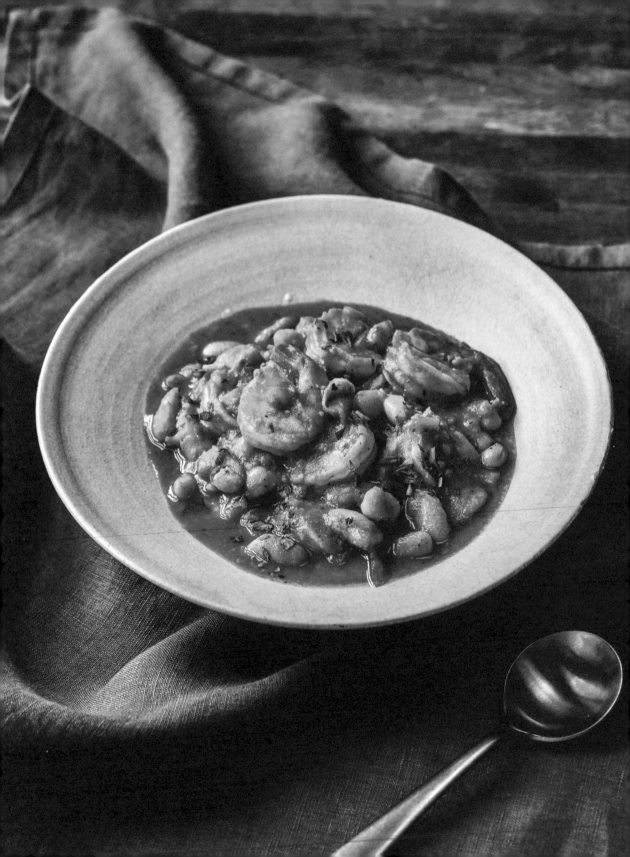

CHILI-GARLIC SHRIMP
WITH CANNELLINI BEANS

An unusual and satisfying dish with contrasting textures and deep flavors, this recipe calls for the best olive oil you can afford. The better the ingredients here, the more they shine. This is equally good served hot or at room temperature, tapas-style. Feel free to make it ahead and relax until dinner.

MAKES 4 SERVINGS

3 garlic cloves

2 fresh red chilies

1 can (19 oz/540 mL) cannellini beans

2 Tbsp flat-leaf parsley

5 Tbsp olive oil, divided

1½ cups/375 mL chopped tomatoes, drained

1 Tbsp tomato paste

1 cup/250 mL chicken stock or Chicken Broth, Traditional-style (page 189)

1 tsp smoked paprika

1 lb/450 g medium shrimp

Salt and pepper

1. Assemble, prepare, and measure ingredients. Mince garlic. Trim and seed chilies. Rinse cannellini beans. Roughly chop parsley.

2. Heat 3 tablespoons of olive oil over medium heat in a large, heavy-bottomed skillet until oil is fragrant but not smoking. Stir in two-thirds of garlic and all the chilies. Stir with a wooden spoon for 1 minute, being careful not to burn garlic. The aroma should be heavenly.

3. Add drained tomatoes and season with salt and pepper. Cook, stirring, for about 5 minutes, or until tomatoes have softened completely.

4. Add tomato paste and cook, stirring, until it has caramelized, about 3 minutes. Stir in beans and stock. Bring to a fast simmer (many little bubbles) and cook until liquid has reduced and thickened slightly, about 4 minutes. Season with salt and pepper.

5. Sprinkle paprika over shrimp and add shrimp and remaining garlic to bean mixture. Simmer until shrimp are opaque and curled into a C shape, about 3 minutes. Drizzle remaining 2 tablespoons of olive oil over shrimp and beans. Taste and adjust seasoning.

6. To serve, divide among four individual bowls and garnish with parsley.

SEARED SCALLOP
AND LENTIL SALAD

Lentils are often a comfort food, but here they are elevated by being dressed
in sesame and ginger, nestled on a bed of greens, and topped with fat, juicy scallops.
Don't be tempted to use red lentils—they cook too quickly and will become mushy.

MAKES 4 SERVINGS

SALAD

½ lb/225 g dried green or
   black lentils
4 garlic cloves
1 bay leaf
5 Tbsp olive oil, divided
3 Tbsp sesame seeds
1 lb/450 g sea scallops
½ lb/225 g mesclun mix
1 oz/30 g arugula
Salt and pepper

SESAME-GINGER DRESSING

1-inch/2.5 cm piece ginger
1 lemon
3–4 Tbsp olive oil
1 Tbsp toasted sesame oil

1. Assemble, prepare, and measure ingredients. Rinse and drain lentils. Peel and smash garlic. Grate ginger. Juice lemon.

2. Bring a large saucepan of unsalted water to a boil over high heat. Turn down heat to medium-low, add lentils and bay leaf, and simmer for 15–20 minutes, or until tender. Drain and transfer lentils to a serving bowl.

3. For the dressing, whisk together ginger, 2 tablespoons of lemon juice, 3 tablespoons of olive oil, and sesame oil. Season with salt and pepper. Add more olive oil, 1 tablespoon at a time, for a thicker consistency. Stir half the dressing into lentils and toss gently. Set aside.

4. In a small skillet over medium-low heat, warm 2 tablespoons of olive oil. Add garlic and stir for about 1 minute. Remove garlic and add sesame seeds, stirring constantly, for about 1 minute or until golden. Be careful not to let them burn. Remove from heat and set aside.

5. Heat 3 tablespoons of olive oil in a large skillet over medium-high heat. Season scallops with salt and pepper, and sear for 2 minutes on each side. Be careful not to overcook scallops or they'll become rubbery.

6. To serve, arrange mesclun and arugula on a serving platter. Mound lentils over top, then place scallops on lentils. Drizzle with remaining dressing and sprinkle with toasted sesame seeds.

CEDAR PLANK TROUT WITH ALMOND AIOLI

For a taste of summer, try this cedar plank technique. It works beautifully on a barbecue, but if you don't have access to one, or the snow is blowing too steadily to consider cooking outdoors, planking in your oven works too. Roasting on cedar planks works with any fish. Cod or halibut are good substitutes for the trout in this.

MAKES 4 SERVINGS

½ bunch flat-leaf parsley

½ cup/125 mL blanched almonds

1 garlic clove

¼ cup/60 mL olive oil

2 Tbsp lemon juice

4 (total weight 1½ lb/680 g) trout fillets

½ tsp cayenne pepper

Salt and pepper

1. Soak one or two cedar planks (you want enough surface area to fit all the trout without crowding) in water for at least 24 hours.

2. Assemble, prepare, and measure ingredients. Finely chop parsley. Preheat oven to 400°F/200°C.

3. In a food processor, pulse almonds and garlic until finely ground. With the motor running, pour in oil, lemon juice, and about ⅓ cup/80 mL of water and combine until mixture is consistency of mayonnaise. Season with salt and pepper. Scrape this aioli into a bowl and refrigerate, covered, until ready to serve.

4. Season trout with cayenne, and salt and pepper. Remove cedar planks from water and place trout skin-side down on top. Place planks directly on oven racks and cook until fish starts to flake, about 10 minutes depending on thickness of your fillets.

5. To serve, remove trout from oven, place on individual plates, and garnish with dollops of aioli and sprinkles of parsley.

SHRIMP AND RADICCHIO SALAD WITH CITRUS VINAIGRETTE

The bright pink shrimp, deep purple-red radicchio, and flecks of green parsley make this dish one of the prettiest in the book. It also tastes good! If you have a grill—or even just a grill pan—try grilling the radicchio instead of oven-roasting it. The slight char from grilling gives the bitter leaves a delicious layer of complexity.

MAKES 4 SERVINGS

SALAD
2 heads radicchio
1 lb/450 g medium shrimp
1 lb/450 g grape tomatoes
2 sprigs flat-leaf parsley
3 Tbsp olive oil, divided
1 Tbsp red wine vinegar
Salt and pepper

CITRUS VINAIGRETTE
1 lemon
6 Tbsp olive oil
2 tsp Dijon mustard
Salt and pepper

1. Assemble, prepare, and measure ingredients. Trim and chop radicchio into large chunks. Peel and devein shrimp. Slice tomatoes in half. Mince parsley leaves. Zest and juice lemon. Preheat oven to 425°F/220°C.

2. For the salad, toss radicchio in a bowl with 2 tablespoons of olive oil and vinegar. Season with salt and pepper. Spread radicchio in a single layer on a baking sheet and roast for 10–12 minutes, until crisp and brown around the edges.

3. While radicchio is roasting, toss shrimp with remaining 1 tablespoon of olive oil. Season with salt and pepper. Place shrimp on a baking sheet, add to oven with radicchio, and roast for 3–5 minutes, or until shrimp form C shapes. Remove shrimp and radicchio from oven and set aside.

4. For the vinaigrette, in a small bowl, whisk together 1 tablespoon of lemon zest, 2 tablespoons of lemon juice, olive oil, and mustard. Season with salt and pepper.

5. To finish the salad, combine radicchio, shrimp, and tomatoes in a large bowl. Add vinaigrette and toss gently to combine. Sprinkle with parsley.

6. To serve, divide among four individual bowls.

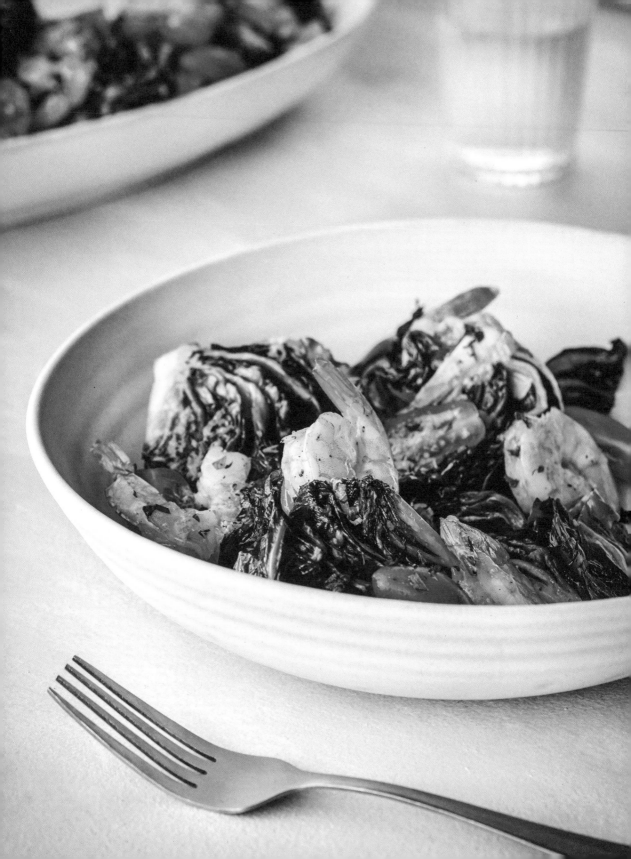

TUNA WITH ZA'ATAR AND TAHINI SAUCE

Za'atar is a mix of spices that originated in the Middle East and is now so popular you can find it in many mainstream grocery stores. But why not make your own? It's another basic recipe to add to your kitchen repertoire: an all-purpose blend you can toss into roasted nuts, over sautéed vegetables, or anywhere you'd use dried herbs.

MAKES 4 SERVINGS

ZA'ATAR

2 Tbsp black or white sesame seeds

1 Tbsp dried thyme leaves

1 Tbsp ground cumin

1 Tbsp ground coriander

1 Tbsp sumac powder

½ tsp salt

¼ tsp Aleppo chili flakes

TUNA

4 (total weight 24 oz/700 g) tuna steaks

3 Tbsp olive oil, divided

6 Tbsp Za'atar, plus more for serving

1 cup/250 mL Tahini Sauce (page 103)

Salt and pepper

1. Assemble and measure ingredients.

2. For the Za'atar, place sesame seeds in a small pan and toast lightly over medium heat for 30 seconds, or until they release their nutty scent. Keep pan moving so sesame seeds do not burn. Let cool in pan.

3. Place sesame seeds, thyme, cumin, coriander, sumac, salt, and chili flakes in a spice grinder or (clean!) coffee grinder. Grind to a fine powder.

4. For the tuna, drizzle fillets with 1 tablespoon of olive oil. Season liberally with 6 tablespoons of Za'atar, and salt and pepper. Heat 2 tablespoons of olive oil in a heavy skillet over medium-high heat until rippling but not smoking. Sear tuna for 2 minutes on each side. Remove from heat and allow to rest for 5 minutes.

5. To serve, place a warm tuna steak on each plate and drizzle with tahini sauce and an extra sprinkling of Za'atar.

PROVENCAL SEAFOOD STEW WITH GARLIC MAYONNAISE

Most culinary traditions have their own variation of seafood stew.
French *bouillabaisse*, Spanish *zarzuela*, San Francisco's American-Italian
cioppino, and Caribbean pepperpot are a few examples. Here,
dried herbes de Provence provide a *soupçon* of the south of France.

MAKES 6 SERVINGS

1 yellow onion

1 fennel bulb

4–6 garlic cloves

1 lemon

½ cup/125 mL olive oil

2 tsp herbes de Provence
(dried thyme leaves,
basil, rosemary, tarragon,
oregano, lavender, and
fennel)

1 tsp chili flakes

½ cup (125 mL) white wine

2 Tbsp tomato paste

4 cups/1 L Fish Broth (page
190) or clam juice

2 cups/500 mL canned plum
tomatoes

2 lb/900 g non-oily fish fillets
(halibut, perch, haddock,
cod)

1 lb/450 g shellfish

6 Tbsp mayonnaise

Saffron (optional)

1 tsp hot sauce

Salt and pepper

1. Assemble, prepare, and measure ingredients. Chop onion. Trim and roughly chop fennel. Mince garlic—you need about 4 tablespoons. Zest and juice lemon.

2. Heat olive oil in a heavy stockpot over medium-high heat. Cook onion, fennel, and 3 tablespoons of minced garlic with herbes de Provence and chili flakes for 12–15 minutes, or until softened completely. Season with salt and pepper.

3. Add wine and tomato paste. Cook until wine has evaporated, about 10 minutes. Add broth (or clam juice) and bring to a boil. Turn down heat to low and simmer, uncovered, for 30 minutes. Strain broth through a fine-mesh sieve into a bowl. Discard residual solids.

4. Return broth to stockpot and set over medium-low heat. Add fish and shellfish and cook for about 5 minutes, or until just opaque or shells have opened. (Discard any whose shells have not opened.) Remove from heat and set aside.

5. In a small bowl, combine mayonnaise with a pinch of saffron (if using), 1 tablespoon of warm water, 1 tablespoon of garlic, 1 tablespoon of lemon juice, 1 teaspoon of lemon zest, and hot sauce. Season with salt and pepper.

6. To serve, scoop fish stew into six individual bowls and garnish with a dollop of garlic mayonnaise. Serve remaining garlic mayonnaise in a small bowl.

FISH PIE WITH POTATO-CAULIFLOWER MASH

To reduce the starchiness of this traditional favorite, use a combination of potatoes and cauliflower, which combine to make a more nutritious mashed topping with fiber and flavor to spare. You can also make this topping with cauliflower only.

MAKES 4 SERVINGS

2 russet potatoes

½ small head cauliflower

4 handfuls spinach leaves

1 yellow onion

2 carrots

4 oz/100 g Cheddar cheese

1 lemon

1 bunch flat-leaf parsley

3 Tbsp olive oil, divided

1 tsp ground nutmeg

1 cup/250 mL heavy cream

1 tsp dry mustard

4 (total weight 1 lb/450 g) cod fillets

Salt and pepper

1. Assemble, prepare, and measure ingredients. Peel and cube potatoes. Separate cauliflower into florets. Chop spinach. Dice onion. Peel and dice carrots. Grate Cheddar. Juice lemon. Chop parsley. Preheat oven to 450°F/230°C.

2. Bring a large saucepan of salted water to a boil and cook potatoes for 10 minutes, or until tender. Add cauliflower and cook for another 5 minutes. Remove vegetables with a slotted spoon, reserving cooking water. Spread veggies out to dry. When they stop steaming, mash with 1 tablespoon of olive oil. Season with nutmeg, and salt and pepper. Set aside.

3. Place spinach in a sieve and pour reserved warm vegetable cooking water over it. When spinach is cool enough to handle, squeeze out any excess water. Set aside.

4. In a skillet over medium-low heat, warm 1 tablespoon of oil. Add onions and carrots and sauté for 5 minutes, or until onions are translucent and carrots are tender. Add cream and bring to a boil for 30 seconds. Remove from heat and stir in Cheddar, 1 tablespoon of lemon juice, parsley, and dry mustard.

5. In a 13- × 9-inch/2 L baking dish, combine spinach and fish. Pour cheese-vegetable sauce over fish and top with mashed potatoes and cauliflower. Brush with olive oil and bake for 20–25 minutes, or until topping is well browned. Remove from oven and allow to rest for 10 minutes. To serve, spoon fish pie onto four plates.

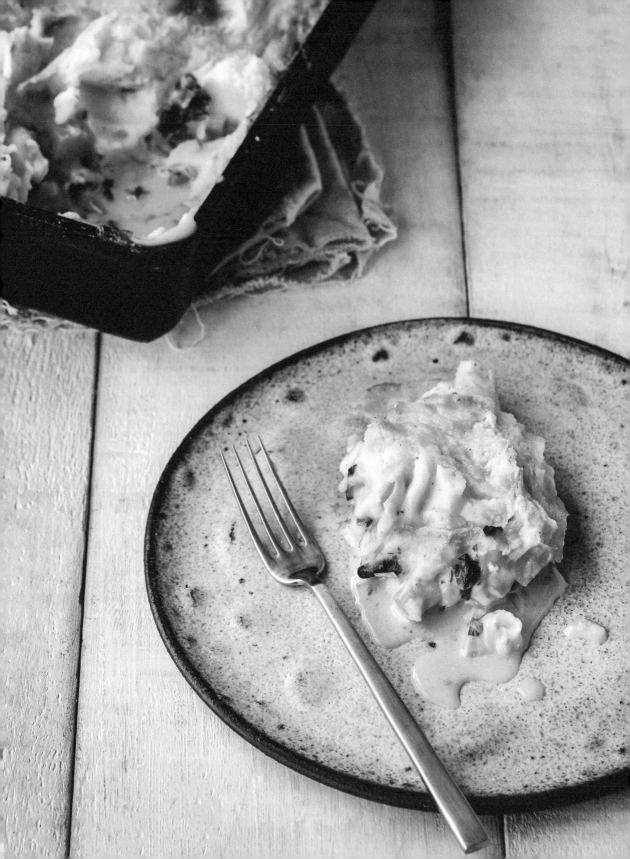

MEATS:
BEEF, LAMB, AND PORK

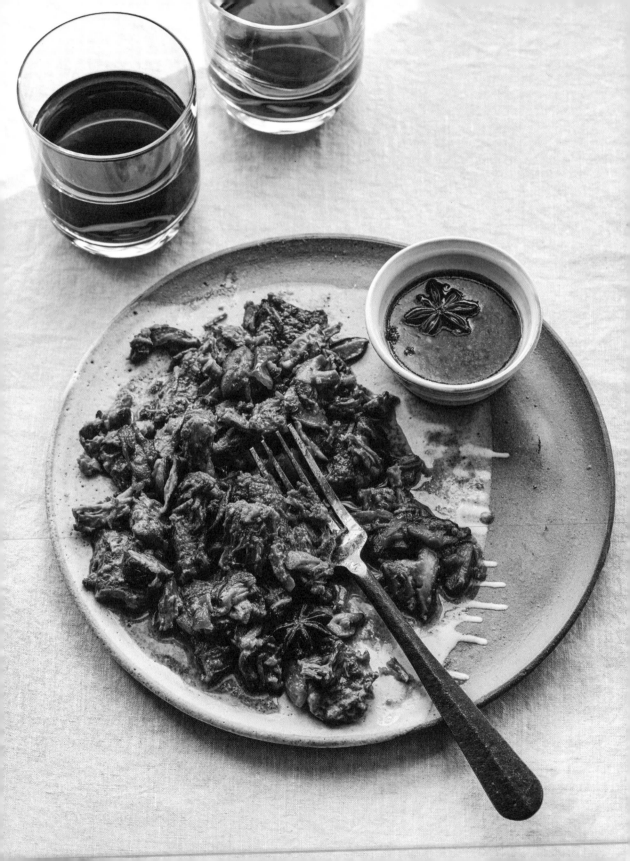

BEEF SHORT RIBS WITH STAR ANISE AND SZECHUAN PEPPER

Get out your slow-cookers and pressure-cookers for this recipe. No matter which cooking method you use, sear the short ribs for a deeper flavor, then braise them slowly to achieve tender beef ribs perfumed with Szechuan pepper, star anise, and cardamom.

MAKES 6–8 SERVINGS

2 yellow onions

3-inch/7.5 cm piece ginger

½ lb/225 g shiitake mushrooms

2 garlic cloves

3 Tbsp olive oil, divided

3½ lb/1.5 kg beef short ribs

2 whole star anise

2 tsp ground Szechuan pepper

1 tsp ground cardamom

1 Tbsp tamari

2 cups/500 mL beef stock or Beef Broth (page 188)

Salt and pepper

1. Assemble, prepare, and measure ingredients. Chop onions. Grate ginger. Slice mushrooms. Slice garlic. Preheat oven to 275°F/135°C.

2. Warm 2 tablespoons of olive oil in a cast iron or enameled cast iron Dutch oven, or other oven-safe pan with a lid, over medium-high heat. Season short ribs with salt and pepper and sear on all sides until deep brown, 15–20 minutes in total. Remove from pan and set aside, leaving residual oil in pan.

3. Add onions, ginger, mushrooms, and garlic to hot oil in pan and sauté for 5–7 minutes, or until onions are translucent. Add star anise, Szechuan pepper, and cardamom. Cook for 30 seconds, stirring constantly. Return short ribs to pan. Stir in tamari and then add just enough beef stock to come up the sides of the meat but not to cover it (you may not need the full 2 cups/500 mL). Cover and braise in oven for 3½–4 hours, until meat is falling off the bone.

4. Transfer ribs to a bowl, pull out and discard bones, and separate meat using two forks. Skim off and discard liquid fat from surface of braising liquid. Bring liquid to a boil over high heat for 8–10 minutes, or until it has thickened and is intensely flavorful. Remove star anise from sauce.

5. Serve short ribs with some of their delicious sauce over top and extra on the side.

COTTAGE PIE
WITH CHEESY MASH

Did you know that shepherd's pie is made with lamb, not beef? We've been calling cottage pie by the wrong name all this time! Potatoes are high in starch, but they help bind the topping in this traditional recipe. You may replace them with cauliflower if you're following a strict low-carbohydrate diet.

MAKES 4 SERVINGS

1½ lb/680 g parsnips or celeriac

½ lb/225 g russet potatoes

1 large yellow onion

1 large carrot

2 sprigs fresh thyme

3 oz/80 g Cheddar or Gruyere cheese

2 Tbsp olive oil

1 lb/450 g ground beef

1 cup/250 mL beef stock

2 Tbsp Worcestershire sauce

1 Tbsp tomato puree

¼ cup/60 mL heavy cream or whole milk

1 Tbsp butter, room temperature

Salt and pepper

1. Assemble, prepare, and measure ingredients. Peel and roughly chop parsnips (or celeriac). Peel and roughly chop potatoes. Dice onion. Dice carrot. Pick thyme leaves from stalks and discard stalks. Grate cheese. Lightly grease an 8-cup/2 L casserole dish with a little butter or olive oil.

2. Bring a medium saucepan of salted water to a boil over medium-high heat, add parsnips (or celeriac) and potatoes, and cook for 15 minutes or until fork-tender. Drain and set aside to dry in colander for 10 minutes.

3. Heat olive oil in a skillet and brown beef thoroughly for 5–7 minutes. Season with salt and pepper. Add onion, carrot, and about 2 teaspoons of thyme leaves. Cook, stirring occasionally, for another 5 minutes, or until onions are translucent and carrots are tender-crisp. Stir in beef stock, Worcestershire sauce, and tomato puree. Lower heat slightly to simmer for 15 minutes.

4. In a mixing bowl, mash parsnips (or celeriac) and potatoes with cream (or milk) and butter. Mix in half the grated cheese.

5. Preheat oven to 350°F/180°C. Pour beef and vegetables into prepared casserole dish, spread mash evenly over top, and sprinkle with remaining cheese. Bake, uncovered, for 30 minutes, or until cheese is nicely browned. Remove from oven and let rest for 10 minutes. Serve in individual bowls.

FLANK STEAK IN
RED WINE DIJON MARINADE

Flank steak is chewier than some cuts of beef but packs so much more flavor.
Because this is a leaner cut, your side dish could emphasize richness:
slaw with crème fraîche dressing, Brussels sprouts with garlic butter, anything
with cheese… Begin this recipe early in the day, or even the day before
you plan to serve it, to give the meat time to marinate.

MAKES 4 SERVINGS

4 garlic cloves
¾ cup/175 mL red wine,
   divided
3 Tbsp Dijon mustard, divided
3 Tbsp olive oil, divided
1½ lb/675 g flank steak
Salt and pepper

1. Assemble, prepare, and measure ingredients. Mince garlic.

2. Combine garlic with ½ cup/125 mL of wine, 2 tablespoons of mustard, 2 tablespoons of olive oil, and salt and pepper. Place steak in nonreactive bowl, pour marinade over top, cover with plastic wrap, and refrigerate for 8–12 hours.

3. Remove steak from marinade, reserving marinade. Pat dry and season meat with salt and pepper.

4. Heat a grill pan over high heat and brush with 1 tablespoon of olive oil. Place steak in pan and grill, turning several times, for 10–12 minutes for medium-rare. Transfer steak to a wooden board, cover loosely with aluminum foil, and allow to rest for 10 minutes.

5. Place reserved marinade in a small saucepan, bring to a boil over high heat, and let bubble away vigorously, without stirring, for 5 minutes. Add the remaining ¼ cup/60 mL wine, return sauce to a boil, and cook for another 5 minutes. Remove from heat and add remaining tablespoon of mustard.

6. To serve, slice steak thinly across the grain and serve with red wine sauce over top.

DELICIOUS MEATLOAF WITH GRUYERE

Making meatloaf is investment cooking at its best. The investment is your time, of course. You're standing at the stove, so why not deliberately create leftovers to enjoy later? This meatloaf has something extra: layers of Gruyere, inside and out. It is equally yummy hot or at room temperature.

MAKES 6–8 SERVINGS

1 lb/450 g Italian pork sausage

1 yellow onion

4 garlic cloves

8 sprigs flat-leaf parsley

3 eggs

1 lb/450 g Gruyere cheese

¼ cup/60 mL sundried tomatoes in oil

2 lb/900 g medium ground beef

1 Tbsp dried oregano

½ cup/125 mL red wine

1 bunch basil

Salt and pepper

1. Assemble, prepare, and measure ingredients. Squeeze sausage meat out of casings. Dice onion. Mince garlic. Chop parsley leaves and discard stalks. In a small bowl, beat eggs just to combine. Grate cheese. Finely chop sundried tomatoes. Preheat oven to 375°F/190°C. Line bottom and sides of a 13- × 9-inch/2 L baking dish with parchment paper or aluminum foil.

2. In a large mixing bowl, use your hands to combine sausage meat and ground beef with onion, garlic, parsley, and oregano. Season with salt and pepper. Add beaten eggs and wine and mix to combine. Spread mixture on a flat surface and pat into a large rectangle about 2 inches (5 cm) thick. Sprinkle three-quarters of the Gruyere, sundried tomatoes, and basil leaves evenly over meat. Roll mixture into a rough cylinder, pinching the ends to seal in cheese.

3. Transfer meatloaf to prepared baking dish, seam-side down, and bake for 1 hour, or until nicely browned. Sprinkle remaining Gruyere over top and bake for another 5 minutes to melt it.

4. To serve, cut meatloaf into generous slices.

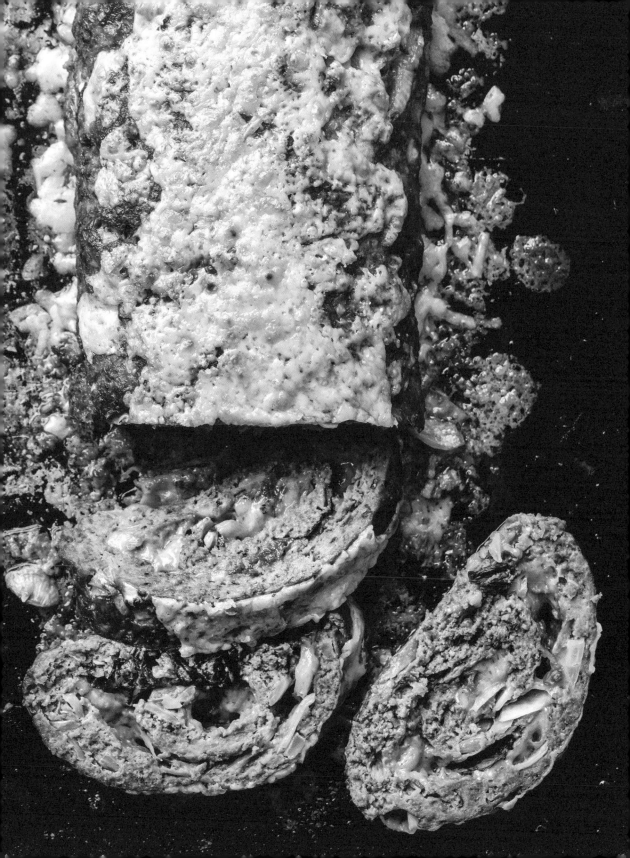

LAMB CURRY
WITH CAULIFLOWER RICE

Cauliflower rice, where have you been all my life? With all the virtues of rice but none of the stodginess, it's a perfect base for curry or chili—or anything you would ordinarily serve over rice. The taste complexity of the curry in this recipe needs the foil of a plain flavor reflector: cauliflower rice to the rescue!

MAKES 4–6 SERVINGS

2 lb/900 g lamb shoulder

2 yellow onions

3 garlic cloves

2 hot green chilies

1-inch/2.5 cm piece ginger

6 large tomatoes

24 oz/700 g cauliflower or prepared cauliflower rice

3 Tbsp ghee or coconut oil, divided

1½ Tbsp garam masala

1½ Tbsp ground cumin

1 Tbsp ground turmeric

1 Tbsp chili powder

2 cups/500 mL coconut milk

2 cups/500 mL chicken stock or Chicken Broth, Traditional-style (page 189)

9 oz/250 g baby spinach leaves

½ cup/125 mL plain yogurt

Salt and pepper

1. Assemble, prepare, and measure ingredients. Cut lamb into cubes and season with salt and pepper. Chop onions. Chop garlic. Chop chilies. Grate ginger; you should have about 1 tablespoon. Chop tomatoes. Pulse cauliflower in a food processor until it resembles grains of rice (unless you're using prepared cauliflower rice).

2. In a large Dutch oven, or other oven-safe pan with a lid, sear lamb in 2 tablespoons of ghee (or coconut oil) until browned all over, 12–15 minutes in total. You may need to do this in batches, depending on the size of your pan, so the lamb doesn't steam. Transfer lamb to a plate and set aside.

3. Place onions, garlic, chilies, and ginger in Dutch oven and sauté over medium-high heat for 3 minutes, or until everything is aromatic and onions are translucent. Be careful not to burn garlic. Add garam masala, cumin, turmeric, and chili powder and stir for about 1 minute to allow spices to bloom. Add tomatoes and stir for a couple more minutes to reduce tomato liquid. Season with salt and pepper.

4. Using a wooden spoon, stir in coconut milk and stock, scraping up any browned bits from bottom of pan, and bring to a boil. Turn down heat to medium, return lamb to pan, and partially cover. Simmer gently for about an hour, or until lamb is very tender.

5. While curry is simmering, in a large skillet with a lid over medium heat, warm 1 tablespoon ghee (or coconut oil). Stir in cauliflower rice and stir to coat well. Season with salt and pepper. Cover, turn down heat to medium-low, and cook for about 5 minutes, or until cauliflower is heated through but not mushy. (Remove pan from heat if lamb hasn't finished cooking by this point.)

6. When lamb is tender, add spinach leaves and swirl in yogurt. Season with salt and pepper.

7. To serve, divide cauliflower rice among four to six plates and top with lamb curry.

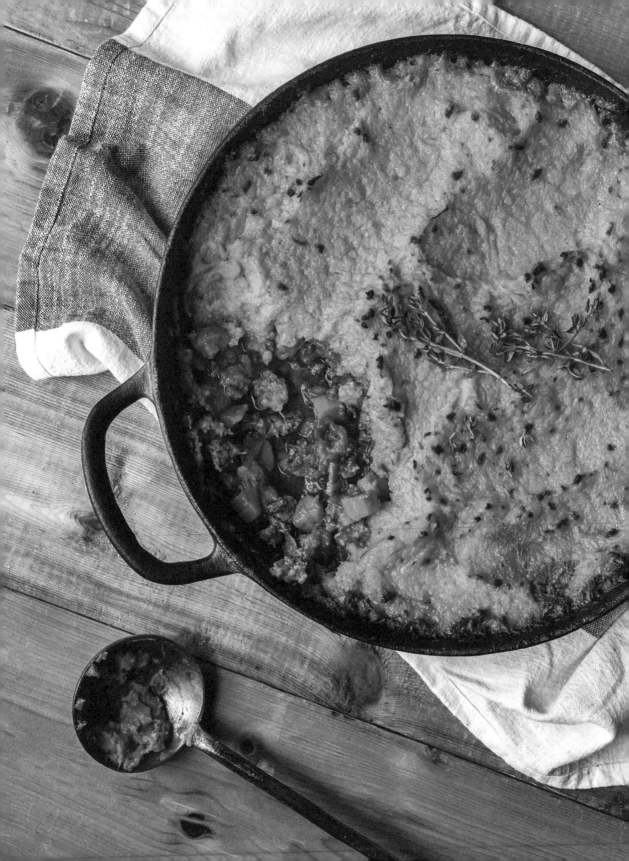

SHEPHERD'S PIE
WITH SWEET POTATO MASH

Here is an authentic shepherd's pie, made with ground lamb. It's also good with a 50:50 combination of beef and pork if you can't find lamb. Instead of the traditional mashed potato topping, I use sweet potatoes, which provide more nutrients and less starch and are a better match for lamb… Go on, try it.

MAKES 4–6 SERVINGS

2 sweet potatoes

4 carrots

1 celery stalk

1 yellow onion

4 slices bacon

3 Tbsp butter

Ground nutmeg

2 Tbsp olive oil

2 bay leaves

1 lb/450 g ground lamb

1 can (14 oz/400 mL) plum
   tomatoes, with juice

1 cup/250 mL chicken
   stock or Chicken Broth,
   Traditional Style
   (page 189)

3 sprigs fresh thyme

1 sprig fresh rosemary

Salt and pepper

1. Assemble, prepare, and measure ingredients. Peel and cube sweet potatoes. Chop carrots. Chop celery. Dice onion. Slice bacon into batons.

2. Bring a large saucepan of salted water to a boil over high heat, add sweet potatoes, and cook for 15 minutes, or until tender. Drain and mash with butter and a pinch of ground nutmeg.

3. While sweet potatoes are cooking, warm olive oil in a skillet over medium heat. Add carrots, celery, onion, and bay leaves and cook for 8–10 minutes, or until onions are translucent and carrots are tender. Add bacon and fry for 5 minutes, or until it has rendered most of its fat but isn't dark brown. Add lamb and cook, stirring occasionally, until nicely browned, about 10 minutes. Add tomatoes with their juice, stock, thyme, and rosemary and bring to a boil. Turn down heat to low and simmer, uncovered, for 20 minutes, or until liquid has reduced by half. Remove and discard bay leaf, thyme, and rosemary. Season with salt and pepper.

4. Preheat oven to 400°F/200°C. Pour lamb mixture into a 13- × 9-inch/2 L baking dish and spread sweet potatoes in an even layer over top. Bake for 25–30 minutes, until bubbling and browned in places.

5. To serve, cut into big squares and place on individual plates.

LAMB KLEFTIKO

This easy and delicious braised lamb recipe will transport you to Kefalonia or Mykonos… or whatever Greek island you daydream about. Start this recipe the day before you plan to serve it to give the lamb time to marinate. Once it's in the oven, pour a glass of ouzo to share with your beloved while your house fills with Mediterranean aromas.

MAKES 6–8 SERVINGS

12 garlic cloves

4 medium parsnips

2 red onions

2 red bell peppers

4½ lb/2 kg lamb shoulder

1 Tbsp olive oil

2 tsp dried oregano

1 tsp ground cinnamon

2 lemons

1 lb/450 g cherry tomatoes

1 bay leaf

Salt and pepper

1. Assemble, prepare, and measure ingredients. Peel and smash garlic. Work 6 cloves into a paste using a mortar and pestle, or a knife and a little olive oil and salt on a cutting board. Peel and chop parsnips. Slice onions. Slice and seed bell peppers. Have ready a large sheet of parchment paper.

2. Place lamb shoulder in a large nonreactive bowl, rub all over with olive oil, and sprinkle with oregano, cinnamon, and salt and pepper. Pat garlic paste all over lamb. Halve one of the lemons and squeeze juice from both halves over lamb. Cover and refrigerate for 8 hours, or up to 12 hours.

3. Preheat oven to 325°F/160°C. In a heavy Dutch oven, or other oven-safe pan with a lid, place remaining 6 garlic cloves, parsnips, onions, bell peppers, tomatoes, and bay leaf. Halve the remaining lemon, squeeze juice over vegetables, and add its peel to pan. Add ½ cup/125 mL water and season well with salt and pepper. Place lamb atop vegetables.

4. Cut a circle of parchment paper to place directly over lamb, large enough to seal it in to cook in its juices. Cover and cook for 4–5 hours, or until lamb is fork-tender. Remove from oven and increase oven temperature to 425°F/220°C. Remove lid from pan.

5. Return pan to oven and cook, uncovered, for 15 minutes, to brown the surface and deepen the flavors. Transfer lamb to a wooden board or platter, cover loosely with aluminum foil, and allow to rest for 10–15 minutes.

6. Return vegetables to oven and cook, uncovered, for another 10–15 minutes, or until nicely browned. Remove from oven and discard bay leaf.

7. To serve, slice lamb thickly or pull it apart into large chunks. Serve on individual plates with the vegetables.

SEARED PORK CUTLETS WITH SAGE AND APPLES

This dish comes together quickly but its elegant presentation suggests otherwise, making it a good choice for a special dinner. Be sure to give the cutlets a good pounding to tenderize them before they are cooked—don't be gentle. I like to sip on apple cider vinegar diluted in really cold water while I cook. Sounds weird, I know, but try it!

MAKES 4 SERVINGS

2 small tart apples

1½ lb/680 g pork cutlets (6–8 cutlets)

6 garlic cloves

2 Tbsp butter

Ground cinnamon

3 Tbsp olive oil, divided

4 anchovies

12 sage leaves

1 Tbsp apple cider vinegar

Salt and freshly ground black pepper

1. Assemble, prepare, and measure ingredients. Core and cut apples into eighths but don't peel them. Pound pork cutlets to ½-inch/1 cm thickness using a meat tenderizer. Peel and smash garlic.

2. In a large skillet over medium-high heat, melt butter. Add apples, season with a pinch of cinnamon and salt and pepper, and cook for 12–15 minutes, turning every so often, until apples have softened but not turned into applesauce. Transfer apples and their cooking juices to a bowl.

3. In the same skillet, cook 1½ tablespoons of olive oil with 3 garlic cloves, 2 anchovies, 6 sage leaves, and a liberal grinding of black pepper for about 30 seconds. Add half the cutlets and cook for 2 minutes per side, until deep brown in places. Transfer cooked cutlets to a platter and keep warm. Repeat with remaining olive oil, garlic, anchovies, sage leaves, and cutlets.

4. Return the same skillet to medium heat, add vinegar, and stir for about 2 minutes to pick up any brown bits from bottom of pan and reduce liquid slightly, just until starting to thicken. Gently stir this mixture into the apples.

5. To serve, arrange pork cutlets on a serving platter. Carefully place apples on top and drizzle cooking juices over everything.

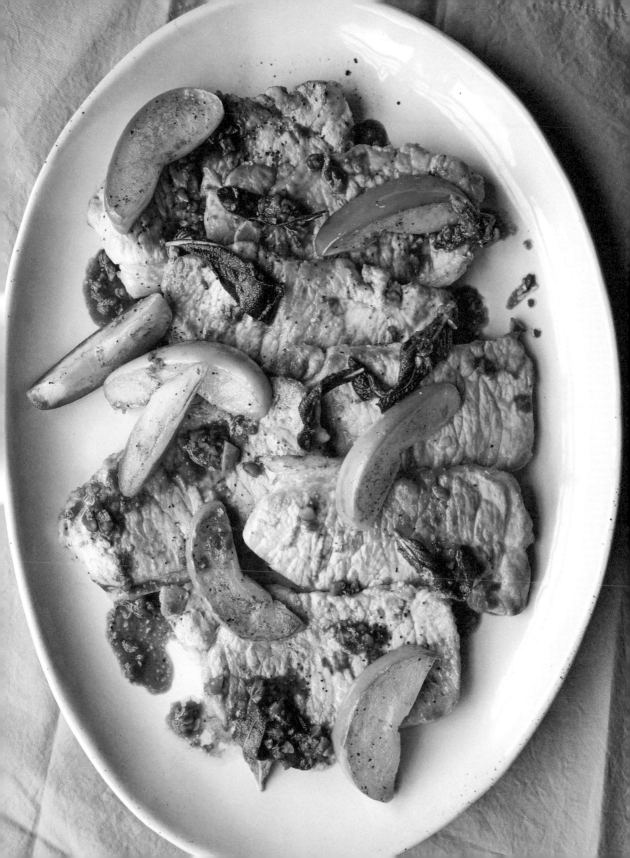

PORK BELLY
WITH STAR ANISE

Braising the pork belly, not submerging it as in a stew, is the key to success in this recipe. Leaving some of the meat exposed above the liquid allows the fat to brown, crisp, and render, making the cooking juices delicious and full of flavor.

MAKES 4 SERVINGS

2 lb/900 g pork belly

1 fennel bulb

3 garlic cloves

4 cardamom pods

1 Tbsp olive oil

4 bay leaves

4 whole star anise

1 Tbsp fennel seeds

1½ cups/325 mL white wine

2–3 cups/500–750 mL chicken stock or Chicken Broth, Traditional-style (page 189)

1 Tbsp wholegrain mustard

Salt and pepper

1. Assemble, prepare, and measure ingredients. Score pork belly skin in a diamond pattern. Season with salt and pepper. Trim and slice fennel. Peel and crush garlic. Crush cardamom in a mortar and pestle. Preheat oven to 350°F/180°C.

2. Warm a roasting pan on the stovetop over medium heat. Add olive oil and then fennel, garlic, cardamom, bay leaves, star anise, and fennel seeds and stir for a couple of minutes until fragrant. Push vegetables and aromatics to the side, add pork, skin-side down, and cook for 8–10 minutes, or until its fat turns a rich brown. Turn pork skin-side up.

3. Add wine to pan to deglaze it, scraping cooked bits from bottom of pan with a wooden spoon but trying not to splash the pork. Bring to a boil, then pour in enough stock to come up to the layer of fat just below the skin. Don't submerge the fat. Place pork in the oven and braise, uncovered, for 2½ hours.

4. Transfer pork belly to a wooden board, cover loosely with aluminum foil, and allow to rest for at least 10 minutes.

5. Skim excess fat from cooking juices with a spoon or turkey baster. Heat remaining juices on stovetop over medium-high heat, whisk in mustard, then taste and adjust seasoning if necessary. Remove and discard bay leaves, star anise, and cardamom. To serve, slice pork and serve on individual plates with extra sauce on the side.

PORK LOIN ROAST
WITH TEA RUB

Tea is an incredibly versatile ingredient, so don't limit yourself to infusing it in water and drinking it. For example, why not add it to recipes as you would any dried herb? It's deeply flavorful, particularly Earl Grey, which is redolent with bergamot. Tea also makes a sophisticated dry rub for pork, chicken, or fish.

MAKES 4 SERVINGS

6 Tbsp loose-leaf Earl Grey tea or Pique Earl Grey crystals
1 Tbsp garlic powder
1 Tbsp onion powder
1 Tbsp olive oil
3 lb/1.3 kg pork loin roast
Salt and pepper

1. Assemble and measure ingredients. Preheat oven to 450°F/230°C. Line a baking sheet with a large sheet of waxed or parchment paper.

2. Combine tea leaves (or crystals), garlic powder, and onion powder and spread over prepared baking sheet. Using your hands or a pastry brush, rub olive oil into pork loin, then roll loin over tea seasoning on baking sheet. Season liberally with salt and pepper.

3. Place pork loin, fat-side up, in a baking dish just large enough to hold it snugly and roast for 20 minutes. Turn down heat to 350°F/180°C and continue to roast for another 40 minutes. Transfer pork to a wooden board, cover loosely with aluminum foil, and allow to rest for 10 minutes.

4. To serve, slice pork and serve on individual plates.

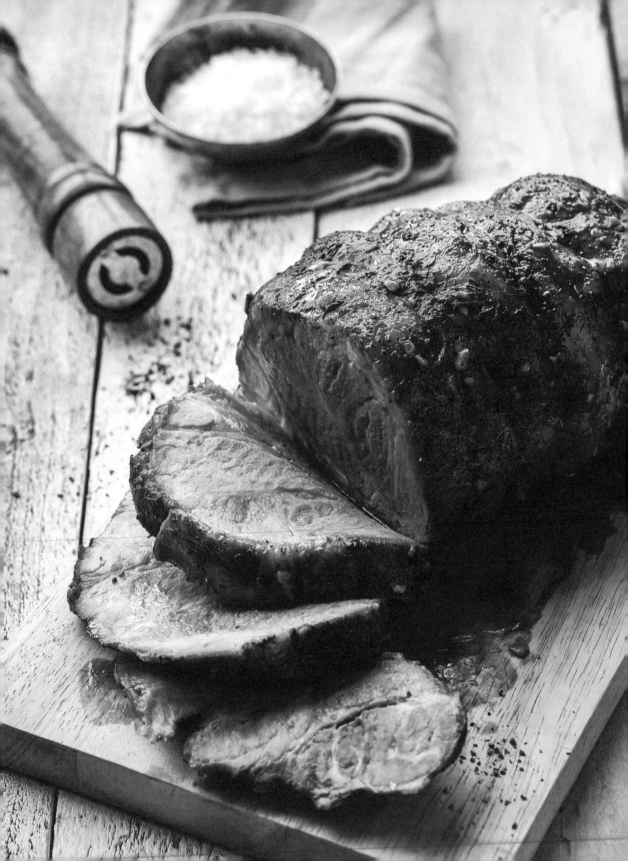

SLOW-ROASTED PORK WITH DIJON AND CHIPOTLE

Appetizing aromas will swirl around your home for hours as this pork roasts.
It's an economical choice, perfect to feed a crowd… or a smaller
gathering with leftovers (hooray!). The roast will be unbelievably tender
and deeply flavored as reward for your patience.

MAKES 6–8 SERVINGS

4½ lb/2 kg boneless pork
   butt or shoulder
2 sprigs fresh thyme
3 garlic cloves
1 tsp ground chipotle pepper
   or smoked paprika
2 Tbsp Dijon mustard
Salt and pepper

1. Assemble, prepare, and measure ingredients. If pork is not
   already tied with kitchen twine, tie it up into a nice little
   bundle. Season generously all over with salt and pepper.
   Place fat-side up in a small roasting pan or baking dish just
   small enough to hold it snugly and allow to come to room
   temperature, about an hour. Pick thyme leaves from sprigs
   and chop. Mince garlic. Preheat oven to 475°F/245°C.

2. In a small bowl, combine thyme, garlic, and chipotle pepper (or paprika) with mustard. Season with salt and pepper.
   Using a pastry brush, coat pork with mustard mixture.

3. Roast pork for 15 minutes, then remove from oven. Turn
   down oven to 200°F/95°C. Cover pork with aluminum foil,
   return to oven, and slow-roast for 8 hours.

4. To serve, slice warm pork thinly and arrange on individual
   plates. Or allow pork roast to cool overnight, covered and
   refrigerated, and reheat, covered, at 250°F/120°C for about
   30 minutes before slicing and serving.

PORK TENDERLOIN WITH FIVE-SPICE AND GINGER-GARLIC SAUCE

The Chinese five-spice in this recipe imparts a taste that is difficult to identify if you're not familiar with the spice but is so appetizing. Because pork tenderloin is a lean cut, the coconut oil in the ginger-garlic sauce is crucial for a silky, satisfying finish.

MAKES 4 SERVINGS

TENDERLOIN

1 tsp garlic powder

1 tsp ground ginger

1 tsp Chinese five-spice powder

2 sprigs fresh cilantro

1½ lb/680 g pork tenderloin

1 Tbsp olive oil

½ cup/125 mL Ginger-garlic Sauce

GINGER-GARLIC SAUCE

1 lime

1 garlic clove

1-inch/2.5 cm piece ginger

½ cup/125 mL tamari

2 Tbsp coconut oil

1 tsp rice wine vinegar

Salt and pepper

1. Assemble, prepare, and measure ingredients. Zest and juice lime. Mince garlic. Grate ginger. Combine garlic powder, ground ginger, and five-spice powder in a small bowl. Pick leaves from cilantro stalks, discard stalks, and chop leaves. Preheat oven to 400°F/200°C. Have ready a large sheet of waxed paper or plastic wrap.

2. For the tenderloin, place waxed paper or plastic wrap on counter and evenly sprinkle dry spice mix over it. Gently roll meat in spice mix. Heat olive oil in a heavy skillet over medium-high heat and sear pork all over, for a total of 4–6 minutes. Leaving any browned bits in skillet, transfer pork to a baking sheet and roast in oven for 12–15 minutes. Remove pork from oven, tent loosely with foil, and allow to rest on baking sheet.

3. For the sauce, combine 1 tablespoon of lime juice, 2 teaspoons of lime zest, garlic, 2 teaspoons of ginger, tamari, coconut oil, and vinegar. Return skillet in which pork was seared to medium-high heat, add about 2 tablespoons of water, and scrape any browned bits from bottom of pan with a wooden spoon. Stir in ginger-garlic mixture and cook to reduce and thicken slightly, about 5 minutes. Set aside.

4. Transfer roasted pork to a wooden board and slice thinly. Divide slices among four plates and drizzle with the sauce.

TREATS AND SMALL BITES

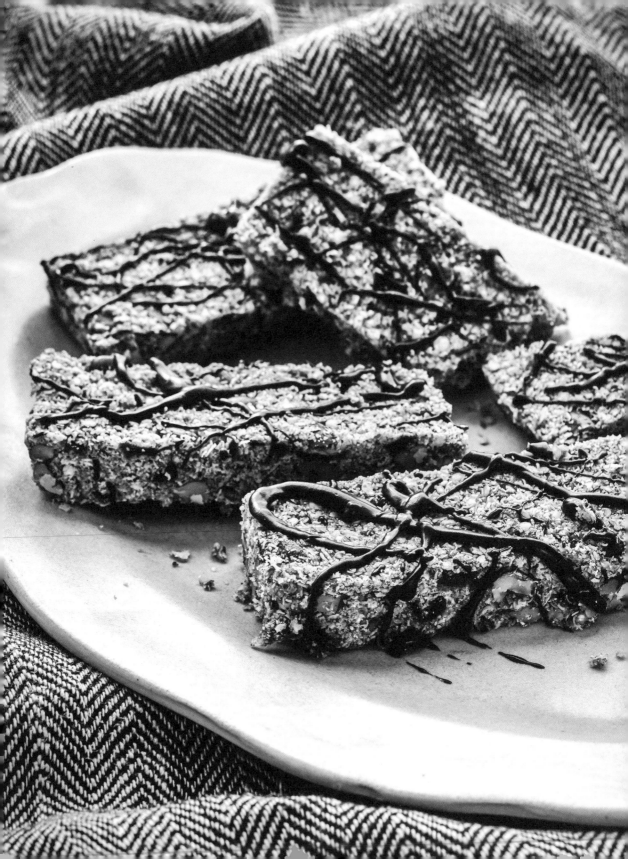

NUT BARS WITH CHOCOLATE DRIZZLE

The original version of this recipe called for maple syrup, but without its overpowering sweetness, the wonderful nut and chocolate combo really shines. Who needs the extra sugar? These are better without it!

MAKES 16–24 BARS

3 oz/80 g raw or roasted almonds, pecans, or walnuts

3 oz/80 g pitted dates

1 egg white

1½ cups/375 mL quinoa flakes

¼ cup/60 mL ground flax

1 tsp ground cinnamon

½ tsp ground nutmeg

¼ cup/60 mL olive oil

4 oz/100 g dark chocolate (70% cocoa)

Salt

1. Assemble, prepare, and measure ingredients. Chop nuts. Chop dates. Beat egg white to soft peaks. Preheat oven to 350°F/180°C. Have ready an 8-inch (20 cm) square baking pan.

2. In a mixing bowl, combine nuts, dates, and egg white with quinoa flakes, flax, cinnamon, nutmeg, pinch of salt, and olive oil. Press into baking pan and bake for 30 minutes, or until firm and golden. Allow to cool in pan for 1 hour.

3. Melt chocolate in a double boiler over low heat, or in a small bowl in the microwave. Drizzle over baked bars and allow to cool completely before you slice into bars and serve. Leftovers will keep at room temperature in an airtight container for up to 3 days.

ALMOND FIG CAKE

For special occasions when a sweet treat is called for, try this traditional almond flour and olive oil cake. It contains no refined grains or refined sugar, only a small amount of pure honey. Check the label to be certain there is no corn syrup in the honey. Garnish with fresh fruit, if you like.

MAKES ONE (8-INCH/20 CM) SINGLE-LAYER CAKE

1 lemon

10 fresh figs

¼ cup/60 mL olive oil

¼ cup/60 mL pure honey

2 large eggs

1½ cups/375 mL almond flour

1½ tsp baking powder

⅛ tsp salt

1. Assemble, prepare, and measure ingredients. Zest and juice lemon. Slice figs lengthwise. Preheat oven to 350°F/180°C. Lightly grease an 8-inch (20 cm) round cake pan and line bottom and sides with parchment paper.

2. In a large mixing bowl, combine 2 tablespoons of lemon juice, 1 tablespoon of lemon zest, olive oil, honey, and eggs. Whisk in almond flour, baking powder, and salt. Pour batter into prepared cake pan and arrange fig slices prettily atop batter. Bake for 30–35 minutes, or until a cake tester or wooden skewer inserted in center comes out clean.

3. Invert onto a plate, then invert again so cake is fig-side up, and slide onto a rack to cool completely.

4. To serve, cut cake into slices and serve on individual plates.

CHICKEN LIVER PÂTÉ

This rich pâté is delicious spread over crunchy vegetable slices—think large bias-cut carrots—or Seedy Crackers (page 181). It is elevated by the addition of brandy, Worcestershire, and hot sauce and has delectable umami.

MAKES APPROXIMATELY 2½ CUPS/625 ML

6 garlic cloves

1 yellow onion

1½ lb/680 g chicken livers

1 Tbsp olive oil

¼ cup/60 mL brandy

1 tsp ground nutmeg

1 Tbsp Worcestershire sauce

2 tsp hot sauce

½ lb/225 g butter

Salt and pepper

1. Assemble, prepare, and measure ingredients. Peel, smash, and chop garlic. Dice onion. Rinse chicken livers under cold water and remove any large external veins. Pat dry with paper towels and set aside on a plate.

2. In a large sauté pan over medium-high heat, warm olive oil. Add garlic and onion and cook, stirring frequently, for 4 minutes, or until brown but not singed. Add chicken livers. Season generously with salt and pepper. Cook, stirring constantly, for 2 minutes to sear livers. Turn down heat to medium-low and cook for 6–8 minutes, or until livers are pink—not red—in the center.

3. Add brandy and nutmeg, using a wooden spoon to scrape up any browned bits from the bottom of the pan. Add Worcestershire and hot sauces, then remove from heat and transfer to a glass or ceramic bowl. Allow to cool for 10 minutes, then cover and refrigerate for 20 minutes, stirring once.

4. Tip chilled chicken livers, garlic, onion, and any collected juices into a food processor or blender. Process or blend to a coarse puree, then add butter, 2 tablespoons at a time, until incorporated. Scrape down the sides between additions. Season with salt and pepper.

5. Transfer pâté to a smallish bowl (about 3 cups/750 mL capacity), cover with plastic wrap, making sure it touches the surface of the pâté, and refrigerate for at least 1 hour and up to 1 week. Allow pâté to come to room temperature before serving.

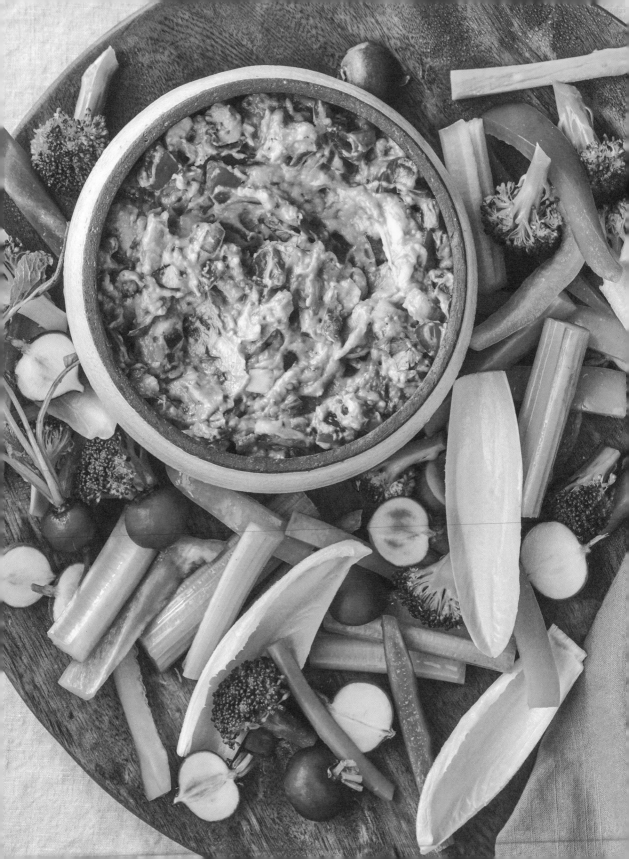

GUACAMOLE WITH CRUNCHY VEGETABLES

This classic dip is raised to new heights with the addition of chunks of tomatoes and red onion. It is delicious served very fresh with crunchy cruciferous vegetables, such as broccoli and cauliflower, but you can blanch them so they're easier to digest, if you prefer. Try not to overmash the avocado or overmix the ingredients—guacamole should not be mushy like baby food.

MAKES ABOUT 2 CUPS/500 ML

3 ripe avocados

2 garlic cloves

1 jalapeño pepper

2 limes

½ lb/225 g grape tomatoes

1 red onion

4 sprigs fresh cilantro

Salt and pepper

VEGGIE SUGGESTIONS:

- Belgian endive: leaves separated
- Broccoli: blanched for 3 minutes
- Carrots: raw, cut into sticks
- Cauliflower: blanched for 3 minutes
- Celery: cut into sticks
- Radishes: halved
- Red and yellow bell peppers: sliced lengthwise into strips

1. Assemble, prepare, and measure ingredients. Halve avocados, discard pits, and scoop flesh into a bowl using a tablespoon. Mince garlic. Seed and mince jalapeño pepper. Zest and juice limes. Chop tomatoes. Finely chop onion. Chop cilantro leaves and stems.

2. In a large bowl, mash avocado coarsely with a fork, so some chunks remain. Stir in garlic, jalapeño, 1 tablespoon of lime zest, 2 tablespoons of lime juice, tomatoes, onions, and cilantro. Taste and add more lime juice if you like. Season with salt and pepper.

3. Spoon guacamole into a serving bowl, or if you make it ahead and plan to serve it later, squeeze some lime juice over top, cover with plastic wrap—pressing plastic right onto the surface of the dip—and refrigerate for up to 4 hours.

4. To serve, arrange vegetables in an artful tumble on a serving platter or tray and serve with the bowl of guacamole sitting alongside.

EGGPLANT HUMMUS

Hummus is often a straight-up chickpea and tahini combo, but it's more interesting with some roasted eggplant. The extra little effort is definitely worth it. Hummus makes a perfectly portable lunch. Prep some raw veggies to dip, and away you go!

MAKES ABOUT 2 CUPS/500 ML

1 can (19 oz/540 mL) chickpeas

4 garlic cloves

1 lemon

2 lb/900 g eggplant

3 Tbsp tahini paste

½ tsp cumin

1 Tbsp olive oil

Salt and pepper

1. Assemble, prepare, and measure ingredients. Drain and rinse chickpeas. Mince garlic. Zest and juice lemon. Preheat oven to 400°F/200°C. Line a baking dish just large enough to hold the eggplant snugly with parchment paper.

2. Prick eggplant(s) in several places with a fork, set in prepared baking dish, and roast for 30–40 minutes, depending on size. The flesh should be translucent and creamy, not firm and white. Remove from oven and let rest in baking dish until cool enough to handle. Scrape flesh into a food processor or blender and discard skin.

3. To the eggplant, add chickpeas, garlic, 2 tablespoons of lemon juice, 1 tablespoon of water, tahini, and cumin. Process until silky smooth. Thin with more water and/or lemon juice, about 1 teaspoon at a time, according to your preference. Season with salt and pepper.

4. To serve, spoon hummus into a bowl or platter with a rim. Drizzle with olive oil and a light sprinkling of lemon zest.

KALE CHIPS

What a way to get your veggies! These are as appealing as potato chips but they're less starchy. It's important to arrange the kale leaves in a single layer to bake or they'll turn out chewy instead of crisp. You can also double this recipe.

MAKES 4 SERVINGS

1 bunch curly or lacinato kale

1 Tbsp olive oil

2 Tbsp nutritional yeast

1 tsp salt

1 tsp cayenne pepper

1. Assemble, prepare, and measure ingredients. Strip kale leaves from stalks, discard stalks, and tear leaves into large pieces. Rinse and drain leaves, and set out on clean tea towels to dry completely. The kale has to be well dried for the chips to be crisp. Preheat oven to 300°F/150°C. Line two baking sheets with parchment paper.

2. In a large mixing bowl, use your hands to rub olive oil into dry kale leaves, coating each piece completely. Sprinkle all over with nutritional yeast, salt, and cayenne.

3. Spread kale in a single layer on each baking sheet, then set them on the top and bottom racks in oven. After 10 minutes, switch positions of trays, and bake for another 10 minutes. Remove from oven and allow to cool for 5 minutes.

4. To serve, carefully pour the chips into a bowl and dig in! They will keep for up to 3 days in an airtight container.

OVEN-ROASTED CHICKPEAS

A small handful of crunchy, savory roasted chickpeas is good as a small bite to break your fast or as an unexpected topping for salads. These also work well tossed into Onion Soup with Emmenthal (page 96) just before serving for some crunch. For more spicy heat, amp up the chipotle and chili powders.

MAKES SEVERAL SMALL HANDFULS

2 cans (each 19 oz/540 mL) chickpeas
2 Tbsp olive oil
1 tsp ground cumin
1 tsp chipotle pepper
1 tsp chili powder
Salt and pepper

1. Assemble, prepare, and measure ingredients. Drain and rinse chickpeas. Dry well on clean tea towels. Preheat oven to 400°F/200°C.

2. In a mixing bowl, combine chickpeas with olive oil, cumin, chipotle pepper, and chili powder. Spread chickpeas on a baking sheet, season with salt and pepper, and roast for 30–40 minutes, stirring occasionally to prevent blackening. Start checking on the chickpeas after 25 minutes. If they overcook, it happens quickly. Remove from oven and allow to cool completely on pan.

3. To serve, throw chickpeas into a bowl and pass it around. Leftovers keep well in an airtight container at room temperature for up to 3 days.

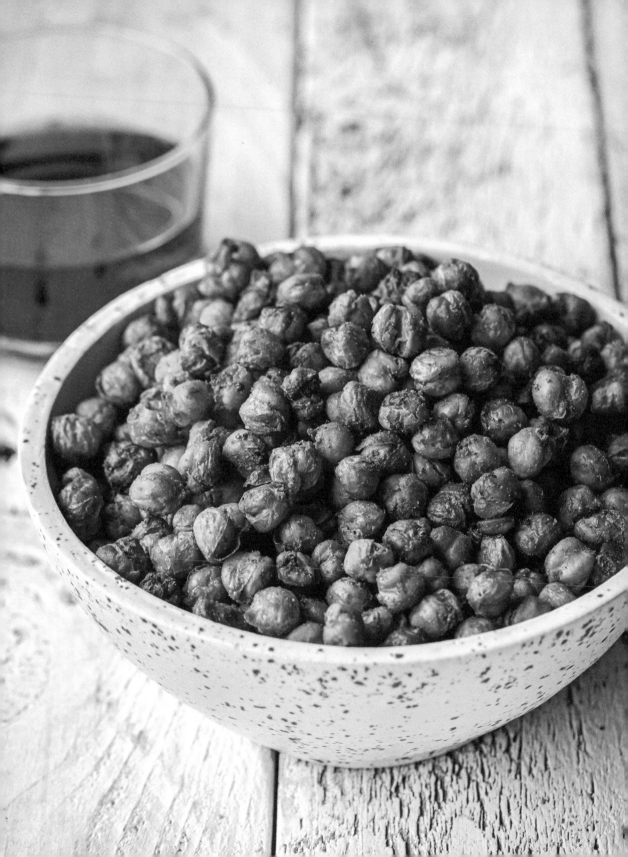

TAMARI ALMONDS

The emphasis in this recipe is on the salty soy taste of the tamari. The tamari almonds available in most specialty food stores tend to be expensive, and you can never be certain they haven't been coated in an unhealthy oil prior to roasting. This is a dry-roast method, resulting in very crunchy, satisfying nuts.

MAKES ABOUT 2 CUPS/500 ML

1 lb/450 g raw almonds
¼ cup/60 mL tamari
1 tsp fresh lemon juice
¼ tsp cayenne pepper
Salt and pepper

1. Assemble and measure ingredients. Preheat oven to 350°F/180°C. Line a baking sheet with parchment paper.

2. In a mixing bowl, toss almonds with tamari, lemon juice, and cayenne. Arrange almonds in a single layer on the baking sheet and roast for 5–7 minutes. Turn off oven and allow nuts to cool for 15 minutes in oven.

3. Remove from oven, season immediately with salt and pepper, and allow to cool completely.

4. To serve, toss almonds into a bowl. Leftovers keep in an airtight container at room temperature for 5 days. (If they get chewy after a few days, reheat for about 5 minutes in 350°F/180°C oven and they'll crisp up.)

WALNUT POWERBALLS

These are great straight from the freezer. Frozen, they're little nut-and-datesicles providing energy, fiber, and protein. They're also yummy chilled, although they're less solid. Eating a couple of these is a good way to break your fast. Powerful, portable, and perfect, they are also a good post-workout snack.

MAKES 24 BALLS

½ lb/225 g roasted walnuts

12 oz/350 g pitted Medjool dates

3½ oz/100 g shredded unsweetened coconut

2 Tbsp coconut oil

1 tsp pure vanilla extract

1 tsp ground cinnamon

½ tsp salt

1. Assemble and measure ingredients.

2. In a food processor fitted with a metal blade, process walnuts with dates, coconut, coconut oil, vanilla, cinnamon, and salt. Roll date-nut mixture into 24 balls and place them in a single layer on a baking sheet. Freeze, uncovered, for an hour to firm them up.

3. Once frozen, transfer balls to an airtight glass container. Refrigerate for up to 1 week or freeze for up to 4 weeks.

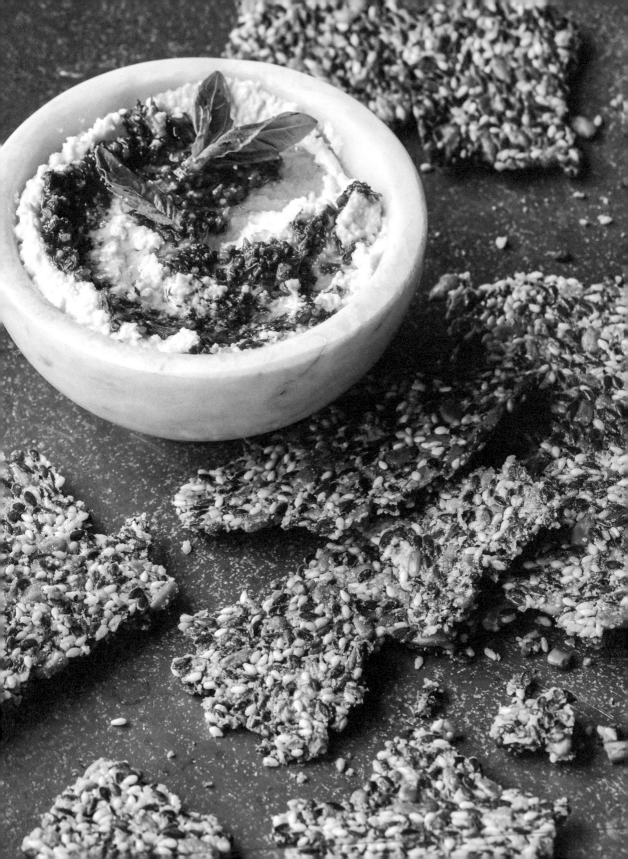

SEEDY CRACKERS

Surprise! Crackers don't have to come from a box; you can make them at home. These are so much better tasting (and better for you) than most commercially made crackers. Since they contain more seeds than flour, they're also more satisfying. And for bonus points, they're sturdy enough for dipping or spreading without crumbling.

MAKES A LARGE SHEET OF CRACKERS

¼ cup/60 mL coconut oil

½ cup/125 mL chickpea flour or almond flour

½ cup/125 mL sunflower seeds

½ cup/125 mL flax seeds

¼ cup/60 mL sesame seeds

Salt and pepper

1. Assemble, prepare, and measure ingredients. Melt coconut oil in a small saucepan over low heat. Preheat oven to 350°F/180°C. Lightly oil a baking sheet.

2. In a mixing bowl, whisk together flour, sunflower seeds, flax seeds, and sesame seeds. Stir in coconut oil and 1 cup/250 mL of boiling water. Using your hands, spread mixture onto the baking sheet, trying to get it as thin and even as possible. Season with salt and pepper, then bake for 30 minutes. Leave oven on.

3. Remove cracker sheet from oven and shake baking sheet or use a metal spatula to loosen. Return to oven and bake for a further 15 minutes. Turn off heat and leave cracker sheet to cool in oven for an hour.

4. To serve, break crisp cracker into whatever size pieces you prefer. Lightly sprinkle with more salt, if you like, and serve.

RICOTTA
WITH PESTO SWIRL

Creamy ricotta with a pinwheel pattern of fresh basil pesto invites you to
dive in with vegetables (try the suggested preparations in Guacamole with Crunchy
Vegetables, page 173) or Seedy Crackers (page 181). Pesto freezes well. It's a
good idea to make a big batch when basil is plentiful in summer and early fall.

MAKES ABOUT 2 CUPS/500 ML

2 big bunches fresh basil

4 garlic cloves

¼ cup/60 mL pine nuts

1 oz/30 g Parmigiano-
   Reggiano or Pecorino

½ cup/125 mL olive oil, plus
   more for serving

1 lb/450 g ricotta

Salt and pepper

1. Assemble, prepare, and measure ingredients. Pick basil leaves from stalks and discard stalks. Poach garlic by immersing whole unpeeled cloves in a small pot of cold water, bringing to a boil over medium-high heat, draining, and repeating once. Slip off skins. Heat pine nuts in a small skillet over medium heat just until golden and aromatic. Grate cheese.

2. In a blender or food processor, combine three-quarters of the basil leaves with poached garlic cloves, pine nuts, and olive oil. Transfer to a bowl and stir in cheese. Season with salt and pepper.

3. Smooth ricotta in an even layer over a serving plate. Swirl in pesto to make a pinwheel pattern. Scatter remaining basil leaves over top and drizzle with some olive oil. Season with more salt and pepper.

SPICY ROASTED NUTS

Nuts are a good choice when you're looking for healthy fat with protein and fiber—
which is what we all should be looking for! This recipe is super simple
and the big-flavored nuts are just right with a glass of red wine. It's a good idea
to keep a batch of these on hand for whenever the urge strikes.

MAKES 2 CUPS/500 ML

1 Tbsp olive oil

2 tsp salt

½ tsp ground cumin

½ tsp ground ginger

½ tsp chili powder

½ tsp cayenne pepper

¼ tsp ground cinnamon

9 oz/250 g raw mixed nuts
(about 2 cups/500 mL)

Salt flakes or coarse crystals

1. Assemble and measure ingredients. Preheat oven to 300°F/150°C. Line a baking sheet with parchment paper.

2. In a large mixing bowl, combine olive oil with salt, cumin, ginger, chili powder, cayenne, and cinnamon. Toss nuts in spice mixture to coat well. Spread nuts in a single layer on lined baking sheet and roast for 10–15 minutes, or until fragrant and dark brown in places. Watch carefully to avoid burning.

3. Remove from oven and allow to cool for 5 minutes on pan before sprinkling lightly with salt flakes or crystals. Let cool completely.

4. To serve, place nuts in a small bowl. Leftovers keep very well in an airtight container at room temperature for up to 2 weeks.

BROTHS AND OTHER BEVERAGES

BEEF AND CHICKEN BONE BROTH

Use any combination of beef and chicken bones to make this broth;
just make sure they weigh 6 pounds (2.7 kilograms) in total.

MAKES ABOUT 3 QUARTS/3 L

2 yellow onions

3 carrots

3 stalks celery

6 garlic cloves

4 lb/1.8 kg chicken bones, wings, necks, backs

2 lb/900 g beef bones, shins or ribs

1 bunch flat-leaf parsley

1 bunch thyme

2 bay leaves

Salt and pepper

1. Assemble, prepare, and measure ingredients. Chop onions, carrots, and celery. Crush garlic.

2. Place bones in a large stockpot and season generously with salt and pepper. Add enough cold water to cover by 2 inches (5 cm). Bring to a boil over high heat, then turn down heat to low and simmer, uncovered, for 1 hour. Skim off any foam that forms on the surface.

3. Add onions, carrots, celery, garlic, parsley, thyme, and bay leaves. Simmer, uncovered, for another 6 hours, continuing to skim any foam from the surface. Remove and discard bones, strain liquid through a fine-mesh sieve into a clean saucepan, and discard remaining solids.

4. Return broth to stockpot, taste, and adjust seasoning with salt and pepper. Pour into a mug to enjoy right away, or keep refrigerated in an airtight container for up to 2 weeks or frozen for up to 4 weeks.

BEEF OR CHICKEN
PRESSURE-COOKER BROTH

For those of you who have a deep and true relationship with your speedy pressure-cooker (Instant Pot, among other brands), here is a variation of bone broth—either chicken or beef—that cooks up in no time and delivers all the yummy goodness of the slower versions.

MAKES ABOUT 2½–3 QUARTS/2.5–3 L

1 yellow onion

2 carrots

2 stalks celery

3 garlic cloves

2 lb/900 g raw beef bones
OR raw chicken wings, feet, and thighs

1 Tbsp apple cider vinegar

1 bay leaf

Salt and pepper

1. Assemble, prepare, and measure ingredients. Chop onion, carrots, and celery. Crush garlic.

2. Place onions, carrots, celery, garlic, bones, vinegar, and bay leaf in a pressure cooker. Season generously with salt and pepper. Add cold water to cover everything by 1 inch (2.5 cm). Cook on high pressure for 3 hours for beef, or 90 minutes for chicken.

3. Remove and discard bones, strain broth through a fine-mesh sieve into a clean saucepan, and discard remaining solids. Return cooked broth to stockpot, taste, and adjust seasoning with salt and pepper. Pour into a mug to sip right away, or keep refrigerated in an airtight container for up to 2 weeks or frozen for up to 4 weeks.

BEEF BONE BROTH

It isn't always easy to find beef bones on display in grocery stores. But ask at the butcher's counter; there will often be bones cut and frozen or ready to be freshly cut for you. Don't be put off by how long it takes to make this broth. You can leave it simmering away while you do other things at home. You'll be so happy to sip on the delicious results!

MAKES ABOUT 8 CUPS/2 L

1 yellow onion

2 carrots

2 stalks celery

4 garlic cloves

3½ lb/1.5 kg beef bones

2 Tbsp apple cider vinegar

2 bay leaves

Salt and pepper

1. Assemble, prepare, and measure ingredients. Chop onion, carrots, and celery. Crush garlic.

2. Place onions, carrots, celery, garlic, and beef bones in a large stockpot and season generously with salt and pepper. Add enough cold water to cover by 1 inch/2.5 cm, followed by vinegar and bay leaves. Bring to a boil over high heat, then turn down heat to low and simmer, uncovered, for at least 10 hours, adding more cold water if necessary to keep bones covered. Skim off any foam that forms on the surface of the broth.

3. Discard bones, strain broth through a fine-mesh sieve into a clean saucepan, and discard remaining solids. Return broth to stockpot, taste, and adjust seasoning with salt and pepper. Pour into a mug to sip right away, or keep refrigerated in an airtight container for up to 2 weeks or frozen for up to 4 weeks.

CHICKEN BROTH, TRADITIONAL-STYLE

This broth is in the style of old-school chicken soup: rich, savory, and good for what ails you. It makes a perfect base for soup and is a delicious clear broth to keep hunger at bay while you're fasting. For a delicious change, use three whole star anise in place of the fresh herbs, and add a tablespoon of tamari to serve.

MAKES ABOUT 3 QUARTS/3 L

1 yellow onion

2 carrots

2 stalks celery

2 garlic cloves

5½ lb/2.5 kg raw chicken bones, wings, feet, neck

2 bay leaves

4 sprigs fresh thyme

1 small bunch flat-leaf parsley

Salt and pepper

1. Assemble, prepare, and measure ingredients. Chop onion, carrots, and celery. Crush garlic. Preheat oven to 450°F/230°C.

2. Place bones in large roasting pan and roast for 45 minutes. Transfer to a large stockpot. Deglaze roasting pan with water, using a wooden spoon to scrape up any brown bits. Pour pan juices over bones in stockpot.

3. Add onions, carrots, celery, garlic, bay leaves, thyme, and parsley and season generously with salt and pepper. Add enough cold water to cover by 1 inch (2.5 cm). Bring to a boil over high heat, then turn down the heat to low and simmer, uncovered, for 2 hours, skimming off any foam that collects on the surface.

4. Discard bones, strain broth through a fine-mesh sieve into a clean saucepan, and discard remaining solids. Return broth to stockpot, taste, and adjust seasoning with salt and pepper. Pour into a mug to sip right away, or keep refrigerated in an airtight container for up to 2 weeks or frozen for up to 4 weeks.

FISH BROTH

In French cooking, this light broth is known as a *fumet*. It has a delicate suggestion of fish flavor and should never be cooked for a long time, as with beef or chicken broth, or it will become too "fishy" and overwhelming.

MAKES 4–6 CUPS/1–1.5 L

2 lb/900 g whitefish bones and heads

2 Tbsp salt

1 small yellow onion

2 garlic cloves

½ fennel bulb

2 stalks celery

1 leek, white part only

1 Tbsp light extra virgin olive oil

1 cup/250 mL dry white wine

2 sprigs fresh flat-leaf parsley

2 sprigs fresh tarragon

1 bay leaf

5 black peppercorns

1. Assemble, prepare, and measure ingredients. Place fish bones and heads in a large bowl, fill with enough cold water to cover bones, sprinkle in salt, and soak bones for 1 hour. Rinse bones in cold water. Dice onion. Crush garlic. Dice fennel. Dice celery. Mince leek.

2. In a stockpot, warm oil over medium heat. Add onions, garlic, fennel, celery, and leeks. Cook, stirring, for 6–8 minutes to soften vegetables, but don't let them brown. Add wine and simmer, uncovered, for 10 minutes to reduce slightly. Add fish heads and bones and enough cold water to cover by 1 inch (2.5 cm).

3. Bring broth to a bare simmer, then add parsley, tarragon, bay leaf, and peppercorns. Turn down heat to low and simmer very gently, uncovered, for 20 minutes.

4. Strain broth through a fine-mesh sieve into a clean saucepan and discard solids. Return cooked broth to stockpot, taste, and adjust seasoning. Pour into a mug to sip right away or keep refrigerated in an airtight container for up to 2 weeks or frozen for up to 4 weeks.

SHRIMP BROTH

This recipe makes a good alternative to Fish Broth (page 190) and it is often easier to acquire shrimp shells than raw fish bones and heads. When you eat shrimp, just toss the shells into a freezer bag and make a broth when you have a good stockpile.

MAKES ABOUT 2 QUARTS/2 L

3 garlic cloves

3 sprigs fresh thyme

2 Tbsp olive oil

Shells of 36–48 shrimp (from about 2 lb/900 g shrimp)

1 bay leaf

Salt and pepper

1. Assemble, prepare, and measure ingredients. Chop garlic. Pick thyme leaves from stalks and discard stalks.

2. In a stockpot, warm olive oil over medium heat. Stir in garlic, thyme, and shrimp shells. Cook, stirring constantly, for about 5 minutes, or until aromatic but not browning. Adjust heat, if necessary.

3. Add enough cold water to cover shells by about 1 inch/ 2.5 cm and toss in bay leaf. Bring to a boil, then turn down heat immediately to low and simmer for 30 minutes. Skim off any foam that forms on top.

4. Strain broth through a fine-mesh sieve into a clean saucepan and discard solids. Return broth to stockpot and season with salt and pepper. Taste broth. If it seems too weak, simmer again until desired flavor is achieved. Pour into mugs and sip hot broth slowly.

BEEF PHO BROTH
AND SOUP

Beef pho is Vietnamese beef soup with garnishes like aromatic herbs, bean sprouts, sliced green onions, and chili peppers that you slip into the hot broth before you eat it. The broth on its own is savory and satisfying, which makes it a good choice during fasting periods, but you can always go the extra step to make the easy and delicious soup for a full meal.

MAKES ABOUT 2–2½ QUARTS/2–2.5 L

BROTH

1 yellow onion

1-inch/2.5 cm piece ginger

4 lb/1.8 kg beef bones, shin and ribs

2 star anise

3 Tbsp fish sauce

Salt and pepper

SOUP

1½ lb/680 g sirloin steak, uncooked, sliced thinly

6 sprigs fresh cilantro

2 green onions, green parts only, sliced thinly

2 cups (500 mL) bean sprouts

1 bunch Thai basil

1. Assemble, prepare, and measure ingredients. Cut onion into quarters. Peel ginger and slice into coins. Preheat oven to 425°F/220°C.

2. Place bones in a single layer on a baking sheet, tuck onion quarters in between bones, and roast, uncovered, for 1 hour, or until onion is dark brown.

3. Transfer roasted bones and onion to a large stockpot. Add ginger, star anise, and fish sauce, season generously with salt and pepper, and add enough cold water to cover by 2 inches (5 cm). Bring to a boil over high heat, then turn down heat to low and simmer, uncovered, for 6 hours. Skim off any foam that forms on surface.

4. Remove bones, strain broth through a fine-mesh sieve into a clean saucepan, and discard remaining solids. Return broth to stockpot, taste, and adjust seasoning with salt and pepper.

5. For the soup, divide steak slices, cilantro leaves, green onions, and bean sprouts evenly among four soup bowls. Ladle very hot broth over top and garnish with a few Thai basil leaves.

TEAS

Tea is made from the plant *Camellia sinensis* and includes black, green,
white, and oolong teas, which differ in their processing, degree of fermentation,
and oxidization. Tea contains antioxidants, which may help to repair tissues.
Green tea also contains catechins, which are believed to suppress appetite. All teas and
tisanes (herbal teas) can be served hot or cold. They can wake you up or relax
you, depending on how long the tea is brewed and how sensitive you are to caffeine.

HERE ARE THE optimal water temperatures and steeping times for the following teas,
whether they are loose-leaf or in bags.

Type of tea	Optimal water temperature	Steeping time
Black	205°F/96°C	3–5 minutes
Green	175°F/80°C	3–5 minutes
Oolong	195°F/90°C	6 minutes
White	185°F/85°C	8 minutes

Pique tea crystals produce instant tea without a lot of chemical additions. Choose
a single variety or combine them. Follow the instructions on the package to make hot or
cold tea. Combined with carbonated water, they make a good substitute for sugary soft
drinks.

TISANES—HERBAL TEAS

If you prefer to avoid caffeine or chemically processed decaffeinated coffee or tea, you may want to try herbal teas. Although they are often called "herbal teas," they are more correctly called "tisanes." Thousands of tisanes are available both loose-leaf and in bags. Do your research, since tisanes are commonly benign but can have medicinal properties: know what the effects can be before you consume. These infusions of leaves, petals, and seeds in hot water can be served hot or cold.

SOOTHING TISANE

8 fresh mint leaves

Bring 1 cup/250 mL water to a boil in a small saucepan. Turn off heat, add mint leaves, and allow to infuse for 5 minutes. Pour into a mug and sip slowly.

DIGESTIVE TISANE

1 oz/30 g fresh ginger

Peel ginger and slice thinly. Bring 1 cup/250 mL water to a boil in a small saucepan. Turn off heat, add ginger, and allow to infuse for 15 minutes.

ALMOND HORCHATA

This refreshing nut-milk beverage originated in Spain and is available widely in Mexico and South America. Variations are consumed in most culinary traditions that incorporate spicy foods. Its cooling effects balance the heat of hot foods, but this is a wonderful drink anytime you need a pick-me-up.

MAKES 4 SERVINGS

4 cups/1 L unsweetened almond milk
4 cinnamon sticks
½ tsp pure vanilla extract, or 1 vanilla bean
1 tsp maple syrup
Ground cinnamon, for serving

1. Assemble and measure ingredients.

2. Combine almond milk, cinnamon sticks, whole vanilla bean (if using), and maple syrup in a saucepan and warm over medium-low heat until milk is steaming. Turn down heat to low and continue to warm for 10 minutes, letting the flavors mingle. Remove milk from heat and discard cinnamon sticks and vanilla bean. If you aren't using a vanilla bean, add vanilla extract now.

3. For hot horchata, serve in four small mugs with a sprinkle of ground cinnamon.

4. For cool horchata, allow milk to cool to room temperature, then refrigerate, covered, overnight. Serve in four glasses with a sprinkle of ground cinnamon.

TURMERIC LATTE

A wonderfully warming drink, this latte will perk up your energy levels—without caffeine. Turmeric is believed to be anti-inflammatory, which can be helpful if you have digestive issues. Experiment with the amount of turmeric until you find the right balance for your taste preferences. The amount listed here is a good starting point.

MAKES 4 SERVINGS

1½ cups/375 mL
    unsweetened coconut milk
1½ cups/375 mL
    unsweetened almond milk
1½ tsp ground turmeric
¼ tsp ground cinnamon
¼ tsp ground ginger
Ground black pepper
Ground cardamom
½ tsp pure vanilla extract

1. Assemble and measure ingredients.

2. Combine both milks with turmeric, cinnamon, ginger, pinch of pepper, pinch of cardamom, and vanilla in a small saucepan over medium-low heat. Whisk well to prevent spices from clumping. Heat until small wisps of steam start to rise.

3. To serve, pour into four mugs and sprinkle with extra cinnamon if you like.

APPENDIX: MEAL PLANS

Sample 7-day meal plan to complement a 16-hour fast

MEALTIME	DAY 1	DAY 2	DAY 3	DAY 4	DAY 5	DAY 6	DAY 7
Morning	**FAST DAY** Turmeric Latte (page 196)	Coconut Pancakes (with berries and cream) (page 56)	**FAST DAY** Green tea	Fried Eggs with Spicy Spinach and Quinoa (page 59)	**FAST DAY** Turmeric Latte (page 196)	Poached Eggs on Spinach with Prosciutto (page 62)	**FAST DAY** Tea or coffee
Midday	Chopped Chicken, Avocado, and Gruyere Salad (page 76)	Burrata, Asparagus, and Radish Salad with Lime Vinaigrette (page 74)	Easy Everyday Omelet (page 55)	Niçoise Salad (page 79)	Eggplant Hummus with veggies (page 174)	Onion Soup with Emmenthal (page 96) Arugula, Fig, and Walnut Salad with Bacon Vinaigrette (page 71)	Thai Vegetable Curry (page 104)
Evening	Cottage Pie with Cheesy Mash (page 148) Grilled Broccoli with Chili-garlic Oil (page 95)	Chicken Thighs with Preserved Lemon (page 109) Pan-roasted Little Tomatoes with Basil Ribbons (page 97)	Scallops with Prosciutto (page 130) Rapini with Chili and Garlic (page 100)	Turkey Chili (page 120)	Lamb Curry with Cauliflower Rice (page 152) Saag Paneer (page 101)	Cod with Mango Avocado Slaw (page 125)	Pork Belly with Star Anise (page 160) Asian Greens with Sesame Oil and Miso (page 88)
Night	Green tea	**FAST DAY** Soothing Tisane (page 194)	Herbal Tea	**FAST DAY** Green tea	Soothing Tisane (page 194)	**FAST DAY** Herbal tea	**FAST DAY** Green tea

Refrain from snacking completely.

Sample 7-day meal plan to complement a 24-hour fast

MEALTIME	DAY 1	DAY 2	DAY 3	DAY 4	DAY 5	DAY 6	DAY 7
Morning	**FAST DAY** Turmeric Latte (page 196)	Berries with Roasted Nuts and Cream (page 54)	**FAST DAY** Tea or coffee	Chia Seed Parfaits (page 53)	**FAST DAY** Turmeric Latte (page 196)	Poached Eggs on Spinach with Prosciutto (page 62)	**FAST DAY** Tea or coffee
Midday	**FAST DAY** Beef and Chicken Bone Broth (page 186)	Burrata, Asparagus, and Radish Salad with Lime Vinaigrette (page 74)	**FAST DAY** Beef and Chicken Bone Broth (page 186)	Niçoise Salad (page 79)	**FAST DAY** Beef and Chicken Bone Broth (page 186)	Onion Soup with Emmenthal (page 96) Arugula, Fig, and Walnut Salad with Bacon Vinaigrette (page 71)	**FAST DAY** Beef and Chicken Bone Broth (page 186)
Evening	Cottage Pie with Cheesy Mash (page 148) Grilled Broccoli with Chili-garlic Oil (page 95)	Chicken Thighs with Preserved Lemon (page 109) Pan-roasted Little Tomatoes with Basil Ribbons (page 97)	Scallops with Prosciutto (page 130) Rapini with Chili and Garlic (page 100)	Turkey Chili (page 120)	Lamb Curry with Cauliflower Rice (page 152) Saag Paneer (page 101)	Cod with Mango Avocado Slaw (page 125)	Pork Belly with Star Anise (page 160) Asian Greens with Sesame Oil and Miso (page 88)
Night	Green tea	**FAST DAY** Soothing Tisane (page 194)	Herbal tea	**FAST DAY** Green tea	Soothing Tisane (page 194)	**FAST DAY** Herbal tea	**FAST DAY** Green tea

Refrain from snacking completely.

Sample 7-day meal plan to complement a 36-hour fast

MEALTIME	DAY 1	DAY 2	DAY 3	DAY 4	DAY 5	DAY 6	DAY 7
Morning	**FAST DAY** Turmeric Latte (page 196)	Berries with Roasted Nuts and Cream (page 54)	**FAST DAY** Tea or coffee	Chia Seed Parfaits (page 53)	**FAST DAY** Turmeric Latte (page 196)	Poached Eggs on Spinach with Prosciutto (page 62)	**FAST DAY** Tea or coffee
Midday	**FAST DAY** Beef and Chicken Bone Broth (page 186)	Burrata, Asparagus, and Radish Salad with Lime Vinaigrette (page 74)	**FAST DAY** Beef and Chicken Bone Broth (page 186)	Niçoise Salad (page 79)	**FAST DAY** Beef and Chicken Bone Broth (page 186)	Onion Soup with Emmenthal (page 96) Arugula, Fig, and Walnut Salad with Bacon Vinaigrette (page 71)	**FAST DAY** Beef and Chicken Bone Broth (page 186)
Evening	**FAST DAY** Beef Pho Broth (page 192)	Chicken Thighs with Preserved Lemon (page 109) Pan-roasted Little Tomatoes with Basil Ribbons (page 97)	**FAST DAY** Chicken Broth, Traditional-style (page 189)	Turkey Chili (page 120)	**FAST DAY** Beef Pho Broth (page 192)	Chili-garlic Shrimp with Cannellini Beans (page 135)	**FAST DAY** Shrimp Broth (page 191)
Night	**FAST DAY** Green tea	**FAST DAY** Soothing Tisane (page 194)	**FAST DAY** Herbal Tea	**FAST DAY** Green tea	**FAST DAY** Soothing Tisane (page 194)	**FAST DAY** Herbal Tea	**FAST DAY** Green tea

Refrain from snacking completely.

Acknowledgments

SPECIAL THANKS TO these cooks for developing, testing, and improving the recipes in *The Obesity Code Cookbook*:

- Carey Broen
- Julia Chanter
- Moira French
- Goody Gibson
- Christopher Jackson
- Charlie Johnston
- David Johnston
- Hannah Johnston
- Alex Mackenzie
- Sandra Maclean
- Diane Morch
- John Morch
- Christine Platt
- Russ Seton

Index